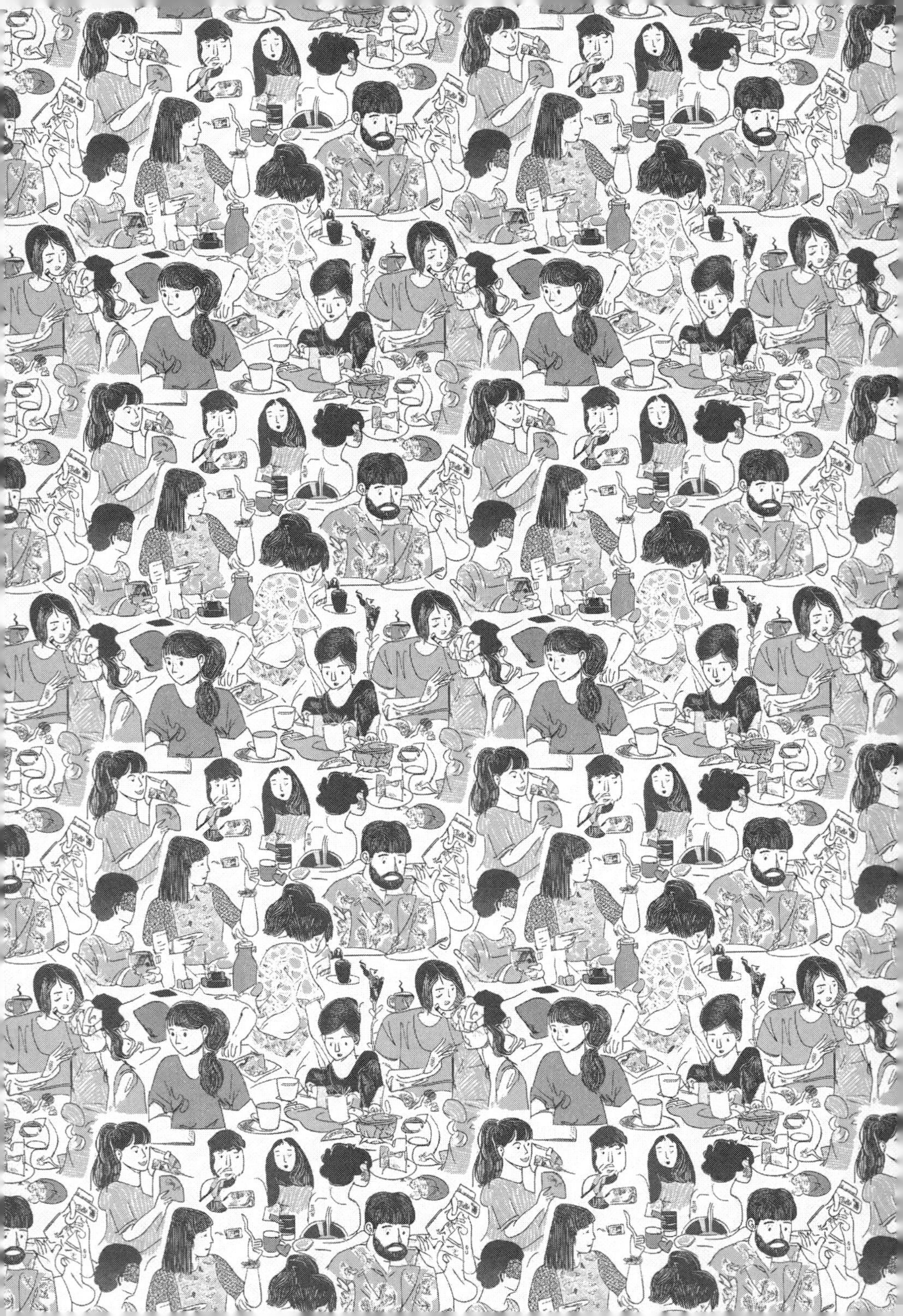

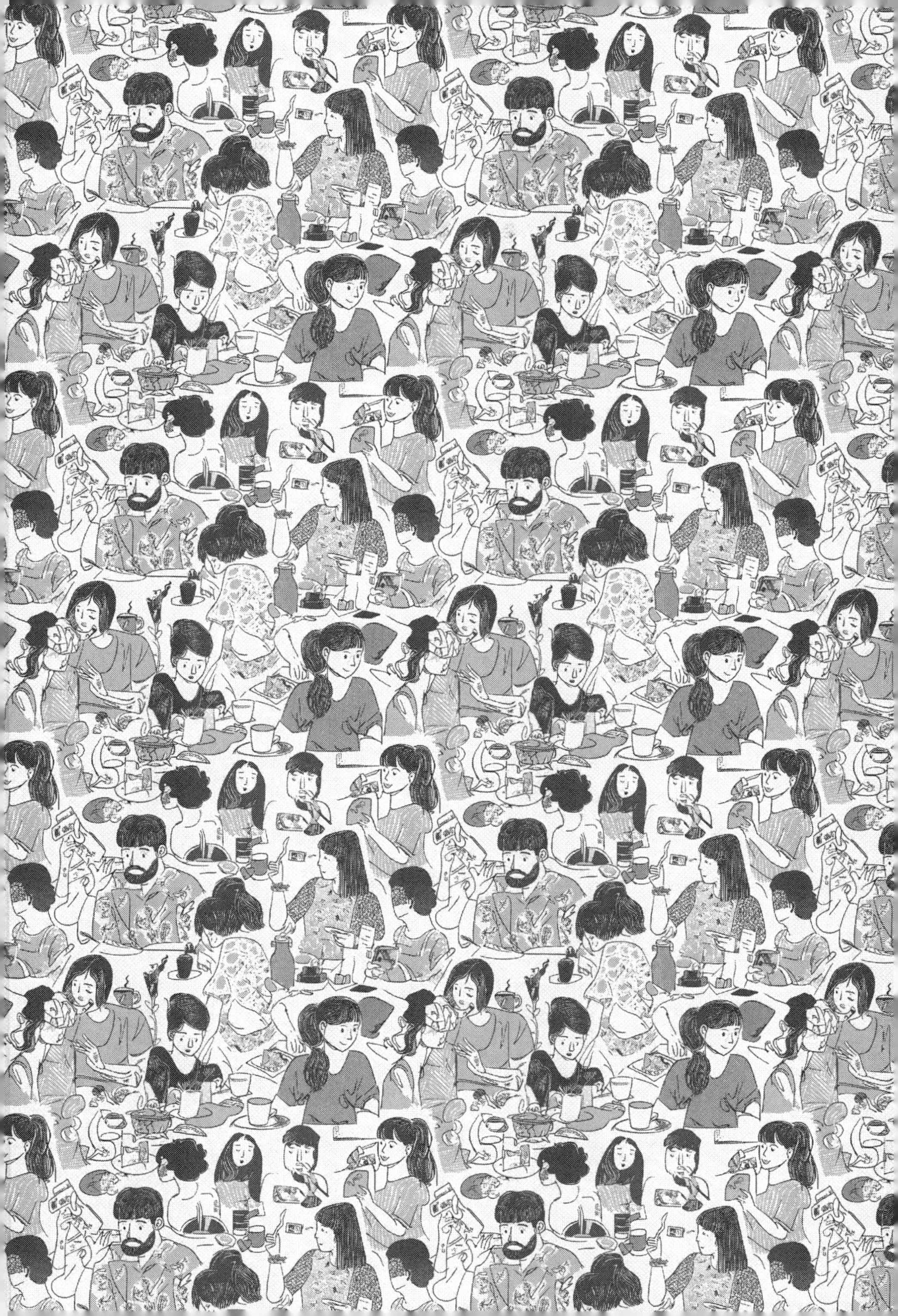

Imprint

Saage Media GmbH
c/o SpinLab
Spinnereistraße 7 - 04179 Leipzig, Germany
E-Mail: contact@saagemedia.com
Handelsregister: Amtsgericht Leipzig, HRB 42755 (Commercial Register: Local Court Leipzig, HRB 42755)
Geschäftsführer: Rico Saage (Managing Director)
USt-IdNr.: DE369527893 (VAT ID Number)

SaageBooks.com//imprint
Publisher: Saage Media GmbH
Publication: 07.2025
Cover Design: Saage Media GmbH
ISBN Softcover (en): 978-3-69141-345-8
ISBN Ebook (en): 978-3-69141-344-1

Legal / Notices

The external links and source references listed in this book were checked at the time of publication. The author has no influence on the current and future designs and contents of the linked pages. The provider of the linked website alone is liable for illegal, incorrect or incomplete contents as well as for damages arising from the use or non-use of the information, not the person who refers to the respective publication via links. All external sources used are listed in the bibliography. Despite careful content control, we assume no liability for the contents of external sources. The operators of the quoted sources are solely responsible for their content. Images and sources from third parties are marked as such. The reproduction, processing, distribution and any kind of exploitation outside the limits of copyright require the written consent of the respective author or creator.
This book has been translated from German. Deviations from the original or translation errors cannot be completely ruled out. All sources linked in the book are available in English. We assume no liability for any content inaccuracies or misunderstandings that may have arisen through translation.
The data in the diagrams that are not explicitly marked with a source are not based on studies but are non-binding assumptions for better visualization.
This book was created using Artificial Intelligence (AI) and other tools. Among other things, tools were used for research, writing/editing, and generating decorative illustrations. Despite careful checking, errors cannot be completely ruled out. We would like to emphasize that the use of AI serves as a supporting tool to provide our readers with a high-quality and inspiring reading experience.
The references contained in this book refer to online sources that have been carefully researched. The information is always reproduced analogously (paraphrasing); literal quotations are avoided. The interpretation and presentation of the reproduced content reflects the opinion of the author and does not necessarily correspond to the intention or opinion of the original authors. When reproducing the meaning, the core statements of the original sources are embedded in the context of this work to the best of our knowledge and belief. Two approaches are used here: Reproduction of meaning: Core statements are paraphrased directly and placed in the thematic context of the book. Transfer and application: Findings from a source that originally came from a different subject area or context are transferred and applied to the specific topic of this book. In both cases, the original formulations and nuances of meaning may differ from the original sources as a result of the transfer, simplification and contextual embedding. The responsibility for the interpretation and the specific application in the context of this book lies with the author. All online sources used are listed in the list of sources at the end of the book. It is recommended to consult the original sources for detailed information, although the permanent availability of online content cannot be guaranteed. The author has endeavoured to present complex issues in a generally understandable way. Simplifications and generalisations cannot be ruled out. No guarantee can be given for the technical accuracy and completeness of the simplified descriptions. The analogous reproduction of findings is carried out conscientiously in compliance with the applicable copyright regulations. When simplifying, transferring and, if necessary, translating content into generally understandable language,

Donar A.I. Saage

Social Psychology: The Basics of Group, Consumer, and Behavioral Psychology

A Practical Guide to Understanding Social Influence, Persuasion, and Interpersonal Dynamics to Navigate Your Social World Effectively.

38 Sources
45 Diagrams
36 Images
9 Illustrations
15 quotes
5 maps

Table of Contents

Additional bonus materials on our website

We plan to provide the following exclusive materials on our website:

- Bonus content and additional chapters
- A compact overall summary
- An audiobook version. (In planning)

The website is currently under construction.

www.SaageBooks.com/social_psychology-bonus-VUR6ZN

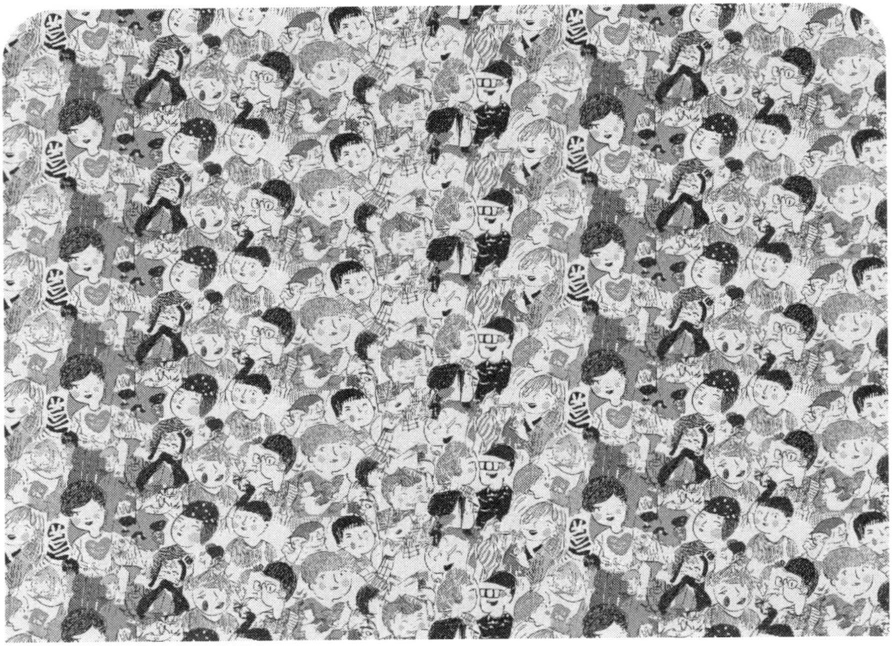

Dear readers,

We sincerely thank you for choosing this book. With your choice, you have not only given us your trust but also a part of your valuable time. We truly appreciate that.

Why do we make certain purchasing decisions? Why do we follow group opinions even when we actually disagree? This book illuminates the psychological mechanisms that govern our behavior in social situations and during consumption. From self-perception to persuasion strategies and group dynamics, the foundations of human interaction are systematically explained. You will learn how cognitive dissonance influences your decisions, the role of authorities and social proof, and how advertising messages affect our subconscious. Practical strategies will help you recognize attempts at manipulation, constructively resolve group conflicts, and make more conscious consumer choices. From analyzing the bystander effect to designing decision-making environments, the content connects scientific insights with concrete applications for professional and everyday life. The book makes the complex relationships between social influence and individual behavior understandable and applicable. Discover the mechanisms that shape your daily actions and develop a deeper understanding of interpersonal dynamics.

This guide provides you with easy-to-understand and practical information on a complex topic. Thanks to self-developed digital tools that also use neural networks, we were able to conduct extensive research. The content has been optimally structured and developed up to the final version to provide you with a well-founded and easily accessible overview. The result: You get a comprehensive insight and benefit from clear explanations and illustrative examples. The visual design has also been optimized through this advanced method so that you can quickly grasp and use the information.

We strive for the highest accuracy but are grateful for any indication of possible errors. Visit our website to find the latest corrections and additions to this book. These will also be incorporated in future editions.

We hope you enjoy reading and discover new things! If you have any suggestions, criticism or questions, we look forward to your feedback. Only through active exchange with you, the readers, can future editions and works become even better. Stay curious!

Donar A.I. Saage

Saage Media GmbH - Team

- www.SaageBooks.com//contact/
- support@saagemedia.com
- Spinnereistraße 7 - c/o SpinLab, 04179 Leipzig, Deutschland / Germany

Quick access to knowledge

To ensure an optimal reading experience, we would like to familiarize you with the key features of this book:

- **Modular Structure:** Each chapter is self-contained and can be read independently of the others.
- **Thorough Research:** All chapters are based on thorough research and are supported by scientific references. The data shown in the diagrams serves for better visualization and is based on assumptions, not on the data provided in the sources. A comprehensive list of sources and image credits can be found in the appendix.
- **Clear Terminology:** Underlined technical terms are explained in the glossary.
- **Chapter Summaries:** At the end of each chapter, you'll find concise summaries that give you an overview of the key points.
- **Concrete Recommendations:** Each subchapter concludes with a list of specific advice to help you put what you've learned into practice.

1. The Social Self: Perception and Influence of One's Own Person

Why do we often behave differently in the presence of others than when we are alone? The self is not a rigid construct but continuously shapes itself through interaction with our social environment. We constantly evaluate ourselves in comparison to others, strategically adjust our behavior to different situations, and grapple with inner contradictions between our beliefs and actions. These processes largely occur unconsciously and yet significantly influence how we see ourselves and how we are perceived by others. The mechanisms behind these everyday phenomena reveal surprising insights into the malleability of our identity.

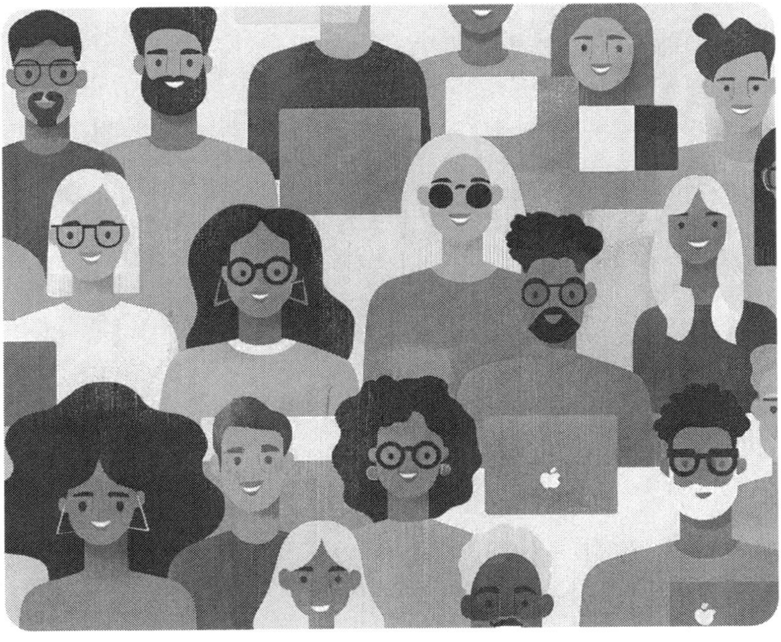

Global Cultures: Individualism vs. Collectivism

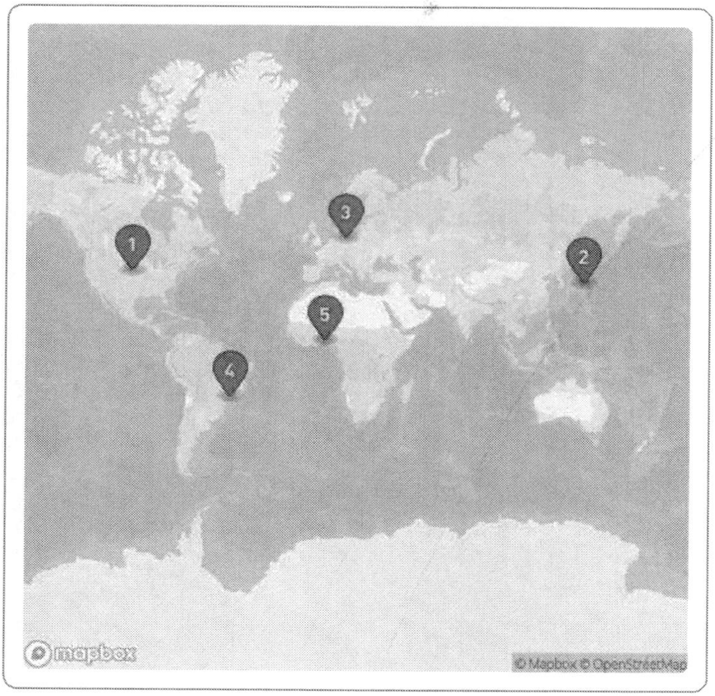

A map illustrating the global spectrum of individualistic and collectivistic cultures, with examples showing how cultural norms shape self-concept and social behavior.

1 **United States**
As a prime example of an individualistic culture, the U.S. emphasizes personal independence, achievement, and self-expression. Self-concept is defined by unique personal traits, and self-esteem is often boosted by individual accomplishments and standing out from the crowd.

2 **Japan**
Japan is a prototypical collectivistic culture where group harmony (Wa) and social roles are paramount. The self-concept is interdependent, defined by relationships and group memberships. Social comparison is often used for self-improvement to better fit in and contribute to the group.

3 **Germany**
Germany represents a form of individualism focused on self-reliance, competence, and directness. While individualistic, there is a strong sense of social order and responsibility, differing from the more competitive individualism of the U.S. Self-esteem is often tied to proficiency and mastery in one's field.

4 **Brazil**
Brazilian culture is strongly collectivistic, especially regarding family and close social circles ('panelinha'). Personal relationships and social networks are crucial for one's identity and success. This coexists with a high value placed on individual expression and enjoyment of life, creating a unique cultural blend.

5 **Nigeria**
Nigerian culture is predominantly collectivistic, with deep emphasis on extended family, ethnic group, and community obligations. An individual's identity is intrinsically linked to their social group. Respect for elders and maintaining one's place within the social structure are key cultural values shaping self-concept.

1. 1 Self-Perception and Social Comparisons

Humans use comparisons with others to evaluate their own abilities, opinions, and status. However, this fundamental process of self-perception becomes a constant challenge in the digital world. Confrontation with idealized life models and seemingly superior individuals distorts one's self-image and often leads to feelings of inadequacy. The inability to consciously manage these comparisons systematically undermines self-esteem and personal satisfaction. Therefore, engaging with the mechanisms of social comparison is not an end in itself. It is the foundation for moving from passive self-devaluation to active self-development.

A mature self-perception does not measure one's worth by the results of social comparisons, but uses a solidified self-esteem as a benchmark to contextualize these comparisons.

"

I have no knowledge of myself as I am, but merely as I appear to myself.

"

Immanuel Kant

Critique of Pure Reason (1781; 1787)
B 158

Kant's statement perfectly encapsulates a central theme of self-perception: the distinction between the 'true' self and the perceived self. In social psychology, our self-concept is understood not as a direct reflection of an inner reality, but as a construct shaped by introspection, feedback from others, and social comparisons. We only know ourselves through the lens of our own subjective experience and how we appear to ourselves in various social contexts, a concept Kant identified as fundamental to human consciousness.

1.1.1 Techniques for Realistic Self-Assessment

A realistic self-assessment does not arise in a vacuum but through a constant comparison with various reference points. The human brain uses comparisons as a fundamental mechanism to categorize its own abilities, traits, and opinions. Often, this process occurs unconsciously and focuses on social comparison, that is, the alignment with other people. In the digital world, this mechanism is perpetually activated by social media. The curated and idealized life designs or body images presented there can lead viewers to feel inadequate. The constant confrontation with seemingly superior others distorts self-perception and can impair psychological well-being by encouraging self-objectification – the tendency to evaluate oneself through the lens of external societal standards [s1]. To develop a more balanced and useful self-view, it is helpful to consciously expand and manage the range of comparison processes.

An effective technique is the **temporal comparison**, where the current self is compared with one's past self or a targeted future self. Instead of asking, "Am I as good as my colleague?", the question here is: "What progress have I made in the last six months?". This perspective shifts the focus from external competition to internal growth. The concrete application involves documenting one's starting point. For example, someone who wants to overcome public speaking anxiety can record their current state and evaluate progress after a period of practice. This creates a fact-based and often encouraging self-assessment that is independent of others' achievements.

Another method is the **dimensional comparison**. Here, a person compares their own abilities and traits across different areas. Instead of a blanket and negative self-assessment, such as "I am unathletic," this approach allows for a more nuanced view: "My endurance is low, but my coordination and flexibility are good." Such an analysis prevents a weakness in one area from dominating the overall self-image. It promotes a realistic assessment of one's strengths and weaknesses and directs attention to existing resources. Practically, this can be implemented by listing various life areas (e.g., career, social relationships, hobbies, health) and separately evaluating one's competencies within these domains.

The **criteria-based comparison** represents a third pillar. In this case, the self is not compared with other people but with a personal, internalized standard or value. Instead of adhering to societal or media-defined notions of success or beauty, the individual defines their own criteria. A person might determine that professional success is not primarily defined by salary and status but by a good work-life balance and meaningful activities. Regular reflection on how one's actions align with these self-imposed criteria leads to a more authentic form of self-assessment.

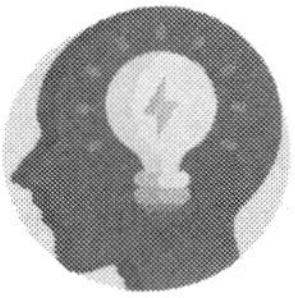

Finally, the **counterfactual comparison**, the contemplation of alternative scenarios ("What if...?"), can be consciously directed. Instead of dwelling in regret over past decisions ("If only I had..."), this technique can be used in a future-oriented manner to learn from mistakes and make better decisions. Reflecting on how an alternative action could have led to a better outcome serves as a learning process for future, similar situations.

These comparison processes are not exclusive but complement each other. By learning to consciously switch between these various comparison standards, one can reduce dependence on often misleading social comparisons. The active choice of the reference frame is thus a manageable tool for achieving a more stable, realistic, and ultimately constructive self-perception [s2].

Good to know

Counterfactual Comparison

The mental simulation of alternative outcomes of past events. Upward-directed thought experiments ('What would have happened if...') can serve learning, while downward-directed alternatives often evoke feelings of relief or happiness.

Criteria-Based Comparison

A form of self-assessment where one's actions and being are measured against personally defined values and goals. This alignment promotes personal autonomy and authenticity, as it is independent of external societal norms.

Dimensional Comparison

The evaluation of oneself by comparing abilities and traits across different life areas. This process fosters a multifaceted self-image and protects self-esteem, as weaknesses in one area can be balanced by strengths in another.

Self-Objectification

A process in which a person primarily views themselves as an object from a third-person perspective. This often leads to increased attention to one's appearance and can push the perception of inner states such as feelings or competencies into the background.

Effectiveness of Self-Assessment Techniques

Comparison of various methods for promoting realistic self-perception

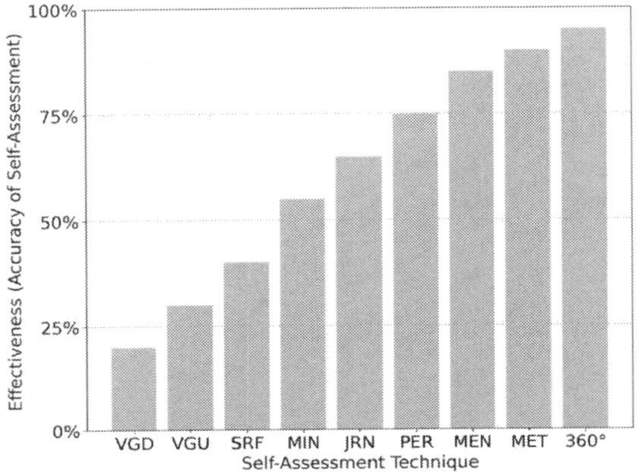

360°: 360-Degree Feedback

MEN: Feedback (Mentor/Expert)

MIN: Mindfulness exercises

SRF: Self-reflection (unspecific)

VGU: Social Comparison (upward)

JRN: Journaling (structured)

MET: Objective metrics (KPIs, grades)

PER: Feedback (Peers)

VGD: Social Comparison (downward)

The diagram clearly shows that techniques based on external and structured feedback exhibit the highest effectiveness for realistic self-assessment. Methods such as 360-degree feedback and the analysis of objective metrics minimize subjective biases and provide a clear picture of one's performance. Obtaining feedback from experienced mentors is also very effective. Pure introspection, such as unspecific self-reflection, is more susceptible to cognitive biases like self-serving bias and therefore less reliable. Social comparisons are particularly ineffective for a *realistic* assessment. Upward comparison often leads to underestimation of one's abilities and demotivation, while downward comparison may boost the ego in the short term but can lead to an unrealistically positive and stagnant self-assessment. The conclusion is that a combination of reflected self-perceptions and, more importantly, validated external feedback is key to accurate self-assessment. The displayed values are estimates intended to illustrate the fundamental mechanisms and relative effectiveness differences of the techniques. They are based on established social psychological concepts.

1.1.2 Constructive Engagement with Social Comparisons

Social comparisons are an integral part of human cognition and cannot be completely avoided. Instead of suppressing them, the key lies in consciously managing and reframing these processes. Constructive engagement begins with understanding the two fundamental directions of comparison: the upward comparison (comparing oneself to individuals perceived as superior in a certain trait) and the downward comparison (comparing oneself to individuals perceived as inferior). While downward comparisons can temporarily boost self-esteem, it is primarily upward comparisons that lead to problems in the digital world. The constant exposure to idealized representations on social platforms can trigger a spiral of dissatisfaction and feelings of inadequacy. The fear of missing out (FoMO) further drives users to expose themselves to such comparisons, which can promote problematic media usage [s3].

A first step towards healthier engagement is recognizing one's own comparison patterns. This can be achieved through mindful self-observation. Ask yourself during or after using social media: Which content or profiles evoke negative feelings such as envy or self-doubt? Becoming aware of these triggers is a prerequisite for actively shaping one's information consumption. This can include muting or unfollowing accounts that consistently provoke negative self-evaluations. At the same time, the focus can be placed on content that inspires without intimidating. Engagement with digitally altered images, including one's own, is negatively correlated with self-esteem and perceived attractiveness. This effect is mediated by self-objectification and comparisons of physical appearance, as they create unrealistic expectations about one's own appearance [s4].

The crucial mental shift lies in reframing upward comparisons. Instead of viewing another person as a rival or a benchmark for one's own failures, they can serve as a source of inspiration or learning. An employee observing a colleague's project success can detach from envy by analyzing not the end result, but the process: What time management techniques were employed? How was communication structured? What specific skills were decisive? This analysis transforms a passive, self-deprecating comparison into an active learning opportunity. The focus shifts from the question "Why am I not as good?" to "What can I learn to achieve my own goals?"

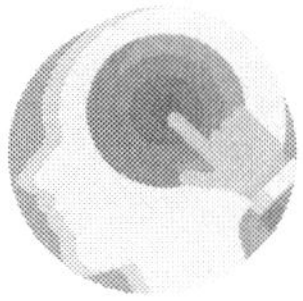

To mitigate the negative emotional effects of comparisons, two complementary attitudes can be cultivated:
- **Focus on Gratitude:** Consciously concentrating on one's own strengths, successes, and positive life circumstances counters the tendency to see only one's deficiencies in light of others' successes. Keeping a gratitude journal can help strengthen this perspective and direct attention to what is already present and positive.
- **Practicing self-compassion:** Social comparisons often lead to harsh self-criticism. Self-compassion means treating oneself with the same kindness and understanding in moments of perceived failure or inadequacy as one would treat a good friend. It acknowledges the human experience of imperfection without falling into self-deprecation.

Ultimately, it is about transforming the comparison process from an automatic, unconscious reaction into a conscious tool for self-reflection and motivation. By recognizing triggers, actively shaping one's environment, and reframing comparison information, the destructive power of social comparisons can be minimized while harnessing their potentially motivating aspect without undermining one's well-being [s3].

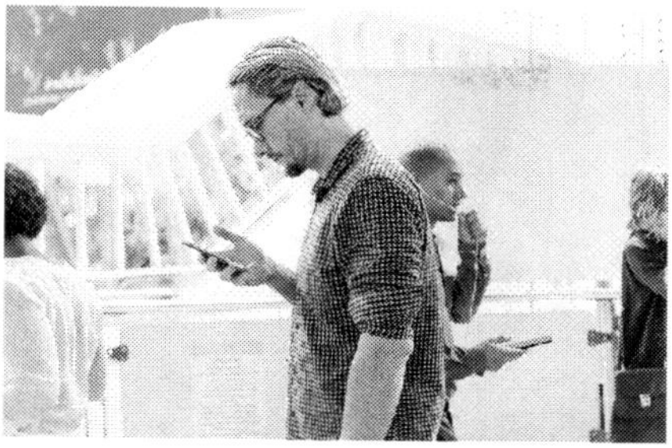

FoMO [i1]

Good to know

Downward Comparison

A form of social comparison in which a person measures themselves against others who are perceived as less capable or worse off in a relevant area. This type of comparison often serves to bolster one's self-esteem and can be used as a strategy to cope with personal setbacks.

Self-Compassion

An attitude that encompasses three essential elements: kindness towards oneself instead of self-criticism, understanding one's own mistakes as part of the shared human experience, and a mindful awareness of one's painful feelings without being overwhelmed by them.

Self-Objectification

A process in which a person begins to see and evaluate themselves from the perspective of an external observer. The body is perceived as an object whose value primarily depends on its external appearance.

Upward Comparison

A process in which a person compares their own abilities or opinions with those of another person who is perceived as better or more successful. This comparison can serve as motivation if the perceived gap seems bridgeable, or lead to negative feelings if the goal appears unattainable.

Social Comparison and Well-being

This chart illustrates the general correlation between the direction of social comparison and its effect on psychological well-being.

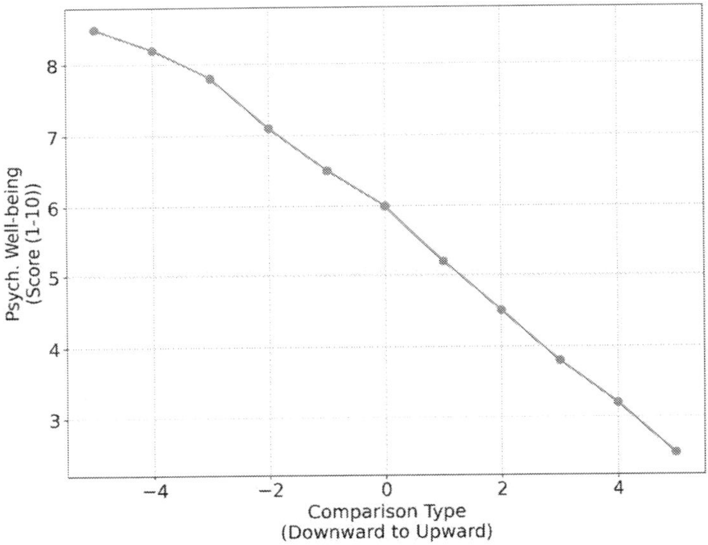

The data shows a clear trend: psychological well-being tends to be higher when individuals engage in downward social comparisons (comparing themselves to those they perceive as less fortunate) and decreases as they engage in upward social comparisons (comparing themselves to those they perceive as superior). Downward comparisons can foster feelings of gratitude and boost self-esteem, while frequent upward comparisons may lead to feelings of inadequacy, envy, and diminished self-worth. It is important to note that these data are estimates intended to illustrate this fundamental principle of social psychology. The actual outcome of any social comparison is heavily influenced by an individual's mindset. A constructive approach can turn an upward comparison into a source of inspiration and motivation, while a non-constructive downward comparison might lead to arrogance instead of gratitude. Therefore, the key lies in consciously managing the comparison process.

1.1.3 The Formation of a Stable Self-Identity in Flux

Self-identity is not a static trait established once in a lifetime, but rather a dynamic structure composed of personal beliefs, values, and self-perceptions. It is in a continuous process of formation and adaptation, driven by new life experiences, changing social roles, and personal development. This process of identity formation is particularly intense during certain life phases, such as adolescence, as personal goals and social affiliations are redefined. Nevertheless, the engagement with one's identity remains a lifelong task. A stable self-identity is characterized not by rigidity, but by the ability to integrate new information and experiences without losing the fundamental sense of continuity and self-worth. It serves as an inner anchor that provides orientation while external circumstances and social expectations change.

Neurobiological research shows that the brain assigns a higher subjective value to concepts perceived as part of one's identity. This is reflected in increased activity in certain brain areas, such as the ventromedial prefrontal cortex (vmPFC), during self-evaluation [s5]. Simply put, what we consider "belonging to us" is valued more highly. This value system influences our behavior and motivation. Actions that align with our self-identity are perceived as rewarding and meaningful, while behaviors that contradict our core beliefs trigger internal resistance or discomfort. Therefore, a stable identity is based on a coherent inner value system that serves as a guideline for decisions. The development of such a system makes a person more resilient to the constant pressure of social comparisons, as the primary measure of self-worth shifts from external to internal.

The consolidation of identity is a process of increasing autonomy from external evaluations. While in early developmental phases, feedback from peers and authority figures strongly shapes self-perception, the focus of a maturing identity shifts to internalized, self-imposed standards [s5]. Instead of primarily aligning one's behavior with what others deem right or successful, it is guided by personally defined values. This does not mean disconnecting from the social environment, but rather developing the ability to filter and evaluate external feedback instead of adopting it uncritically. A person with a solidified identity can accept recognition from others without being dependent on it and reflect on criticism without it shaking their entire self-image.

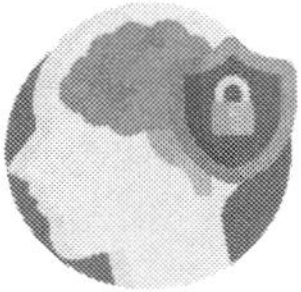

A practical approach to fostering a robust identity lies in recognizing its multifaceted nature. Identity is not a monolithic block but consists of various facets or partial identities. A person is not only their profession but also a partner, friend, athlete, or creative individual. The conscious nurturing of these different life areas creates a resilient self-concept. A setback or crisis in one area, such as losing a job, does not necessarily impair the entire self-esteem. Stability arises from the sum and balance of the parts. If a person loses their professional role, a strong awareness of other life areas—such as skills in a hobby, reliability in friendships, or roles in the family—can maintain the sense of worth and continuity. A helpful exercise is to identify these various roles and the associated positive traits and abilities and to regularly reflect on them.

- **Professional Identity:** What skills and achievements distinguish me in my work life?
- **Social Identity:** What kind of friend or family member am I? What values do I live in my relationships?
- **Personal Identity:** What are my interests and passions outside of obligations? Where do I find meaning and joy?
- **Physical Identity:** How do I treat my body? What do I do for my health and well-being, regardless of external beauty ideals?

This differentiated perspective protects against over-identification with only one life area and the associated risks. The development of a stable identity in flux is thus an active process of self-reflection and conscious alignment with a multifaceted and value-based self-image. It enables flexible responses to life changes while maintaining a consistent sense of who one is.

Good to know

Adolescence

A developmental phase in which social comparisons with peers particularly influence one's self-perception and the search for a personal identity. During this time, social roles and group affiliations are intensely tested.

Coherence

Refers to the feeling of consistency and internal connection of one's beliefs and self-perceptions. A high level of coherence in the self-image helps to process contradictory feedback from the social environment without questioning one's identity.

Internalization

The process by which external norms, values, or beliefs from the social environment are adopted into one's self-concept and become a fixed part of personal conviction.

Over-identification

The excessive attachment of one's self-worth to a single life area, such as profession or a social role. This makes a person particularly vulnerable to negative social comparisons and criticism in that specific area.

Partial Identity

Refers to the various roles and affiliations of a person that together form the entire identity. The conscious nurturing of multiple partial identities can stabilize self-esteem when one is threatened by social comparisons or failure.

Components of Self-Identity

Estimated contribution of different life domains to an individual's overall identity.

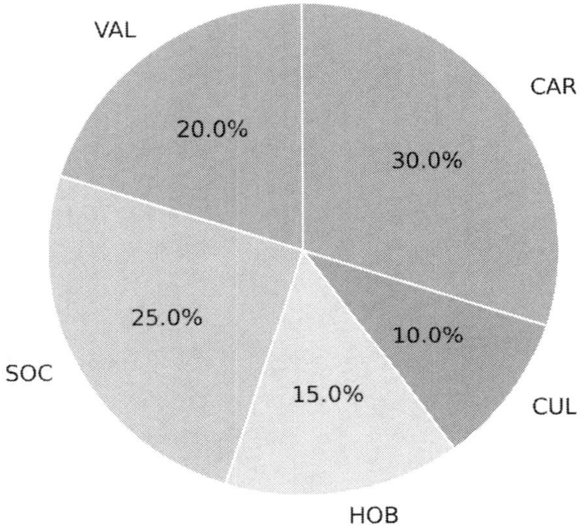

CAR: Career and Work
HOB: Hobbies and Interests
VAL: Personal Values and Beliefs
CUL: Cultural and Group Affiliation
SOC: Social Relationships

This chart illustrates the estimated composition of an individual's self-identity, breaking it down into key life domains. It's important to note that these percentages are illustrative estimates designed to represent a general principle, as the actual composition of identity is highly individual and can fluctuate over a person's lifetime. The chart suggests that professional life ('Career and Work' at 30%) and personal connections ('Social Relationships' at 25%) form the largest components for many people. However, internal factors like 'Personal Values and Beliefs' (20%) are also fundamental, acting as an inner compass. 'Hobbies and Interests' (15%) and 'Cultural and Group Affiliation' (10%) are also significant, highlighting the importance of leisure, self-expression, and a sense of belonging to a larger community. The model underscores that a stable identity is not monolithic but a multifaceted construct, drawing strength from a variety of sources.

1. 2 Self-Presentation and Impression Management

Every person manages the impression they make on others. This intentional self-presentation, also known as impression management, is crucial for social and professional success. It allows one to be perceived as competent, likable, or trustworthy. This creates a constant tension between the desire for authentic behavior and the necessity to adapt to social contexts. An exaggerated performance appears untrustworthy and leads to inner distance. Conversely, a lack of adaptation can jeopardize social acceptance and professional goals. This chapter provides the psychological tools to master this challenging balance with confidence.

Successful impression management is not a departure from authenticity, but rather its strategic application: the conscious decision of which facet of the true self is most effective in a given context.

"Clothes make the man. Naked people have little or no influence on society."

Mark Twain

More Maxims of Mark (1927) edited by Merle Johnson

This witty aphorism directly addresses the core of impression management. Twain humorously points out that outward appearance and self-presentation ('clothes') are crucial for establishing social standing and influence. In social psychology, this aligns with the concept that individuals strategically manage their appearance and behavior to shape how others perceive them, thereby influencing social outcomes.

1.2.1 Strategies for Conscious Self-Presentation

Strategies for conscious self-presentation encompass deliberate actions through which an individual manages the impression others form of them. This process, known as impression management, is programmatic in nature and aims to create, position, and maintain a specific, favorable image of oneself [s6]. It involves a conscious selection and emphasis of individual traits to be perceived as valuable, competent, or otherwise desirable by a target audience. The entirety of these actions shapes a personal brand, which signals an implicit promise regarding the qualities and behaviors of the individual [s6].

A tension often arises in the implementation of these strategies between the desire for authenticity and the necessity of an idealized representation. In the digital realm, particularly on social media, this phenomenon becomes especially evident. Public presentation is often deemed successful when it is perceived as authentic, entertaining, and self-assured [s7]. Authenticity serves as a key factor for positive perception. Simultaneously, actors in this field report an internal conflict: the fear of negative feedback or direct comparison with others leads them to adjust their presentation and show less of their perceived "real" personality [s7]. The presented authenticity is thus often a strategically planned and carefully curated construct.

The idealized component of self-presentation is reflected in the targeted optimization of one's presentation. The use of tools such as image editing software is not only an expression of insecurity but is often motivated by a professional aspiration to create aesthetically pleasing and high-quality content [s7]. This form of self-staging operates in a sensitive area between highlighting positive traits and misleading the audience. The line is thin, as an overly idealized representation can undermine the credibility built once it is exposed as inauthentic.

For effective and sustainable self-presentation, an approach that integrates various considerations is advisable. A technician wishing to position themselves as an innovative expert at a professional conference will highlight different aspects of their personality and knowledge than in an informal meeting with colleagues. Their strategic task is to select those facets that best convey their core message—in this case, competence and future orientation.

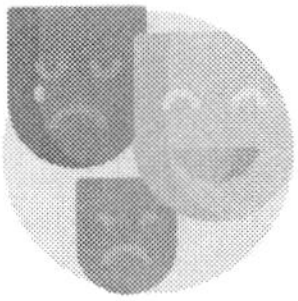

For practical implementation, the following guidelines may be useful:

- **Clarification of the Core Message:** First, one should identify their strengths, values, and unique traits that need to be communicated. This forms the foundation of the personal brand and the promise to the respective audience [s6]. The question is not "Who am I in my entirety?" but "What aspect of my identity do I want to convey in this specific situation?".
- **Striving for Consistency:** The chosen traits should be conveyed uniformly across various channels and interactions to build credibility and reliability. Contradictions between the online profile and personal behavior can quickly damage the carefully constructed image.
- **Balance of Authenticity and Role:** Instead of striving for an unattainable "complete" authenticity, it is more effective to practice sincere role fulfillment. This means remaining genuine and tangible within the chosen strategic orientation without disclosing aspects that are irrelevant or disadvantageous for the context.

Successful self-presentation can lead to an individual being perceived as a role model. This perception carries a responsibility to use one's reach and influence constructively, whether for knowledge dissemination or promoting social causes [s7]. The conscious shaping of one's impression is thus not an act of deception but a continuous process of self-reflection and communication that seeks to balance personal goals with the expectations of the social environment.

Good to know

Consistency

Refers to the coherence of one's behavior and communication over time and across situations. A consistent presence makes it easier for others to form a stable and reliable image of the person and to trust them.

Construct

Refers to a conceptual or social creation that does not objectively exist in reality but is perceived as real through mutual agreement. One's public identity is often such a construct made up of selected information.

Personal Brand

The sum of the impressions that an individual leaves on others. It arises from the conscious and unconscious communication of values, skills, and personality traits with the aim of establishing a clear and recognizable image in the perception of others.

Self-Staging

Describes the process by which an individual shapes their behavior and appearance as if on a stage to achieve a specific effect. This includes verbal and non-verbal signals that are deliberately employed to convey the desired self-image.

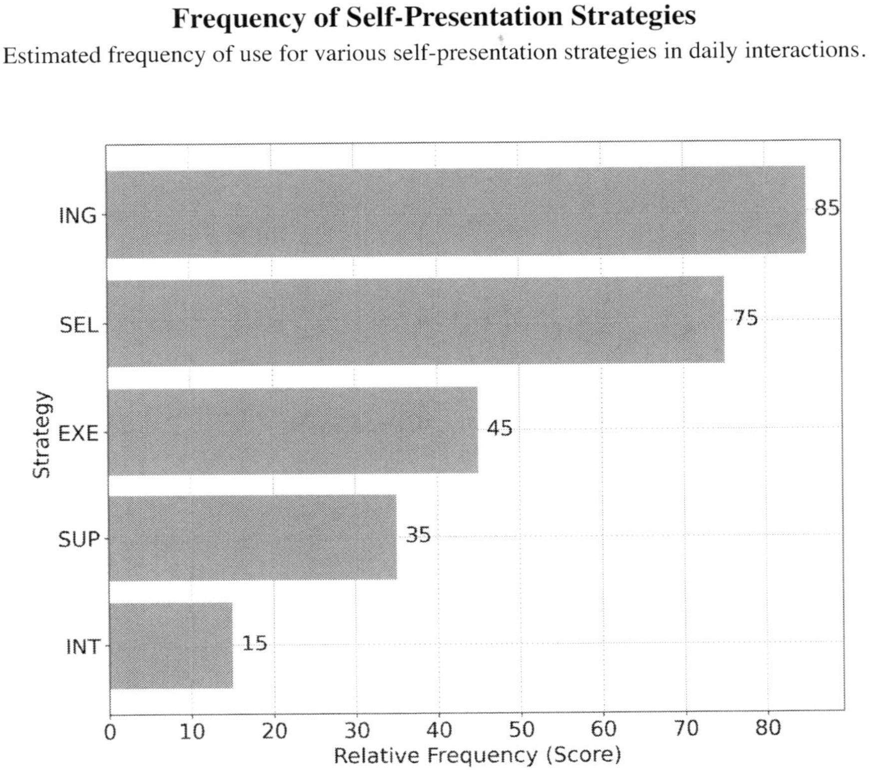

EXE: Exemplification
INT: Intimidation
SUP: Supplication
ING: Ingratiation
SEL: Self-promotion

The chart illustrates that strategies aimed at fostering positive social bonds and demonstrating competence are most common. 'Ingratiation' (e.g., using compliments to be liked) and 'Self-promotion' (e.g., highlighting one's skills) are frequently used tactics in both personal and professional settings. In contrast, strategies like 'Exemplification' (appearing morally superior) and 'Supplication' (presenting oneself as helpless) are employed more situationally. 'Intimidation' is the least common strategy, likely due to its high social risk and potential to damage relationships. It is important to note that these values are reasoned estimates designed to illustrate general principles, as the actual frequency of use heavily depends on individual personality and the specific social context.

1.2.2 Maintaining Authenticity in Social Interaction

A continuous and rigid control of one's image in social situations is associated with cognitive and emotional effort. This constant self-monitoring, aimed at maintaining a specific image, can lead to an inner distance. The individual acts primarily out of concern for how they are perceived by others, rather than from an inner impulse or conviction. This can diminish the sense of being able to shape one's own life autonomously. When external expectations dictate actions, the impression may arise that one is losing control over their social behavior, which can negatively impact overall life satisfaction [s8].

The discrepancy between the presented self and inner experience also carries the risk of social isolation. Although a person may be surrounded by others, they may not feel truly understood or seen, as interactions are based on a carefully constructed facade. Genuine social connection, however, arises through mutual resonance and the sharing of authentic feelings and thoughts. A persistent, strategic self-presentation hinders this exchange and can thus amplify feelings of loneliness, even amidst social activity [s8]. Maintaining authenticity in interaction does not mean revealing every inner state unfiltered. Rather, it is a process of consciously aligning one's behavior with personal values and current feelings, even within the confines of a professional or social role.

The first step in preserving authenticity is sharpened self-awareness. This involves regularly pausing and reflecting on one's feelings, needs, and boundaries in a given situation. Before entering a conversation or social situation, it can be helpful to briefly ask oneself: "How do I feel right now?", "What is important to me in this interaction?" and "Where are my boundaries?". This inner clarification creates a foundation from which one can act without completely disconnecting from their own sensations. It is about maintaining a connection to one's inner state while navigating the social space.

Building on this, authentic behavior can be specified by orienting oneself to core values. Instead of trying to simulate a particular personality, one can focus on choosing actions that align with their deepest beliefs. For instance, a leader who values transparency and teamwork but is naturally more reserved does not need to mimic a loud, dominant leadership style. They can authentically fulfill their role by conducting well-structured meetings, actively listening, and justifying decisions clearly and understandably. Their behavior is then not an imitation but an expression of their values within professional requirements. The actions feel congruent to the individual and are perceived by others as sincere and reliable.

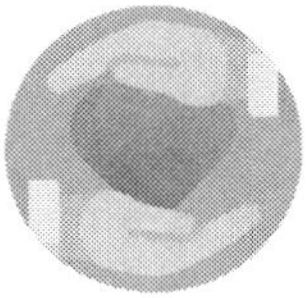

For practical implementation, the following considerations can bridge the inner experience and outer actions:

- **Congruence of verbal and nonverbal communication:** Ensure that your body language, facial expressions, and tone of voice support what you are saying. Incongruences, such as smiling while expressing criticism, can be confusing and diminish credibility. A coherent overall picture emerges when nonverbal signals authentically underpin the verbal message.
- **Courage for measured openness:** Authenticity is strengthened when one is willing to acknowledge uncertainties or human fallibility at appropriate moments. Admitting not knowing an answer immediately or having made a misjudgment on a project does not necessarily weaken one's position. On the contrary, it can build trust and foster collaboration, as it makes the person approachable and human.
- **Setting boundaries as an expression of self-respect:** The ability to respectfully say "no" or communicate one's needs is a strong expression of authenticity. It signals that one values themselves and their resources. This creates clarity in relationships and prevents one from bending out of mere compliance or fear of rejection.

Ultimately, lived authenticity is not a state of complete openness but a dynamic balance. It is the ability to know and maintain one's identity while adapting to the diverse contexts of social life. It enables deeper connections, strengthens the sense of self-efficacy, and thus directly contributes to a more fulfilling social experience.

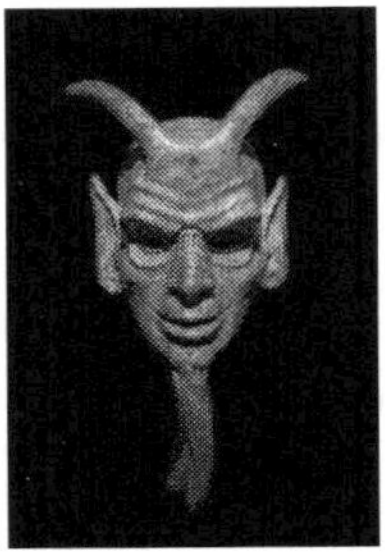

Image [i2]

Good to know

Congruence

Refers to the consistency between the various communication channels of a person. Congruence is particularly noted when verbal statements and nonverbal signals such as body language and tone of voice send a unified and non-contradictory message.

Discrepancy

A perceived contradiction or gap between two aspects of the self, for example, between actual behavior and personal values or between private self-image and publicly presented image.

Facade

A metaphorical term for the carefully controlled and often superficial self-image that a person presents to others. This 'facade' serves to maintain a desired image and conceal true feelings, uncertainties, or intentions.

Image

The deliberately crafted image that a person wishes to convey in public or in social groups. It is the result of conscious or unconscious actions aimed at how one is perceived by others.

Authenticity

Refers to the alignment of a person's external behavior with their inner values and feelings. A person is perceived as sincere when their actions are seen as an expression of their true self.

Components of the Presented Self

Estimated breakdown of the factors influencing our behavior in typical social interactions.

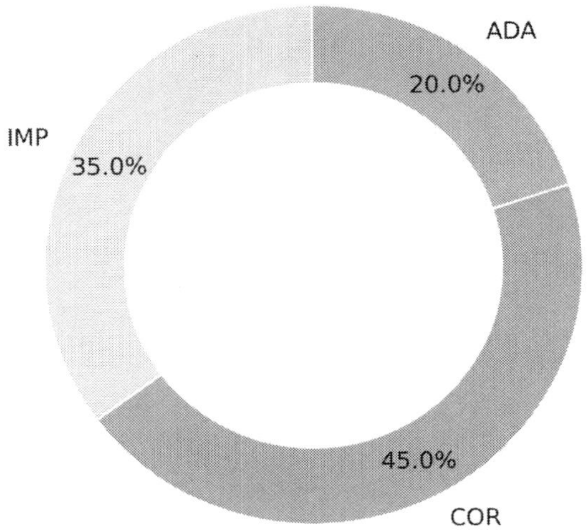

- ADA: Situational Adaptation
- COR: Core Self / Authenticity
- IMP: Impression Management

This chart illustrates the complex interplay of factors that shape our self-presentation. These figures are principled estimates designed to demonstrate the dynamics at play. The largest component, the 'Core Self,' suggests that a significant part of our behavior is driven by a genuine desire for authenticity. However, 'Impression Management' is also a substantial factor, highlighting that we consciously and unconsciously shape others' perceptions to achieve social goals, such as being liked or appearing competent. The 'Situational Adaptation' component, while smaller, is crucial, showing that we constantly adjust our behavior to fit social norms and specific contexts. The key takeaway is that authenticity in social interaction is not the complete absence of management or adaptation, but rather a healthy balance where our core self remains the primary driver of our actions.

1.2.3 Adapting One's Appearance to Social Contexts

The adaptation of one's appearance to different social contexts is a fundamental mechanism of human interaction. People modify their behavior, language, and even their outward appearance to meet the norms and expectations of a specific situation. This process is not a sign of a lack of personality, but rather a form of social competence that enables successful navigation in various environments and the achievement of goals. The ability to recognize situational expectations and adjust one's behavior accordingly is referred to in social psychology as self-monitoring. Individuals with a high degree of this trait act like social observers, flexibly adapting their behavior to the target audience and context to ensure smooth and positive interactions.

The core of this adaptive performance lies in the conscious selection of those facets of one's identity that are most beneficial for the respective context. It is not about playing a foreign role, but about highlighting the appropriate aspects of the authentic self. The vocabulary and topics of conversation during a job interview fundamentally differ from those at an informal gathering after work. In the former case, precise technical terms and a formal address are used to signal competence. In the latter case, a casual language and more personal topics foster social cohesion. The person remains the same, yet the presented side of their personality is strategically aligned with the respective goal—be it professional recognition or social connection. This flexibility allows for building bridges to different people and avoiding misunderstandings that could arise from contextually inappropriate behavior.

Successful adaptation requires a careful analysis of the social environment. Before entering a situation, it is useful to decode the prevailing codes. This includes, among other things, dress codes, hierarchical structures, communication styles, and taboo topics. In a creative startup, a casual dress style may express a spirit of innovation, while in a conservative law firm, a formal suit signals seriousness and respect. Consciously aligning one's appearance with these conditions facilitates social acceptance and the building of trust.

However, excessive or purely reactive adaptation also carries risks. When behavior is almost exclusively driven by the perceived expectations of others and the connection to one's own values and beliefs is severed, it can lead to a feeling of alienation. The person then acts like a chameleon that changes its color but seems to lack a stable core. Such over-adaptation, where the individual feels they are merely reacting to external stimuli rather than acting actively, can undermine the subjective expectation of being able to influence one's life circumstances. The impression of losing control over one's social actions arises because the actions no longer stem from an inner stance but from a compulsion to conform.

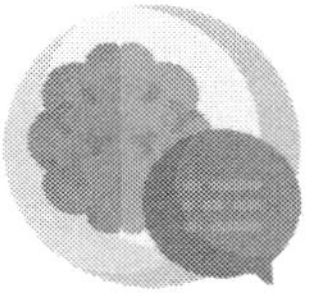

To avoid these pitfalls, a structured approach can help that considers both situational demands and personal integrity:

- **Situation Analysis:** Capture the unwritten laws of the environment. Observe how successful actors communicate and present themselves in this context. What topics are discussed, what tone prevails, and how formal or informal is the interaction?
- **Goal Definition:** Clarify for yourself what impression you want to convey in this specific situation. Should your competence, creativity, trustworthiness, or approachability be in the foreground? Your goal determines which facets of your personality you emphasize.
- **Behavior Adjustment:** Adapt specific aspects of your appearance. This may involve choices regarding clothing, the volume of your voice, your word choice, or your body language. An upright posture and direct eye contact can convey confidence in a business meeting, while a more relaxed body posture signals openness in a creative brainstorming session.

Mastery in adapting to social contexts thus lies in balance. It is the art of being flexible enough to be effective in diverse social arenas while remaining steadfast enough to preserve the core of one's identity. Context-sensitive self-presentation is not self-neglect but an expanded form of communication based on respect for the other and a clear understanding of one's own goals.

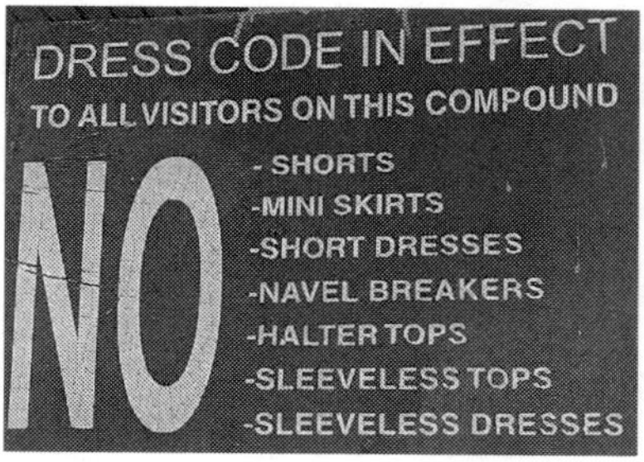

Dress code [i3]

Good to know

Personal Integrity

The alignment between one's values, beliefs, and actual behavior. A person with high integrity acts consistently according to their inner principles even under social pressure.

Self-Monitoring

A personality trait that describes the extent to which a person adjusts their behavior to external situational factors. Individuals with high self-monitoring change their appearance depending on the audience, while those with low self-monitoring exhibit more consistent behavior across different situations.

Social Acceptance

The positive reception and recognition of a person by a group or society. It is a fundamental human need and a common motive for adapting one's behavior to social norms.

Social Competence

The ability to act effectively and appropriately in social situations to achieve personal goals while maintaining positive relationships with others. It includes, among other things, empathy and the skill to correctly interpret verbal and nonverbal signals from others.

Impression Management in Social Contexts

Degree of self-presentation in various social contexts and its relation to social success.

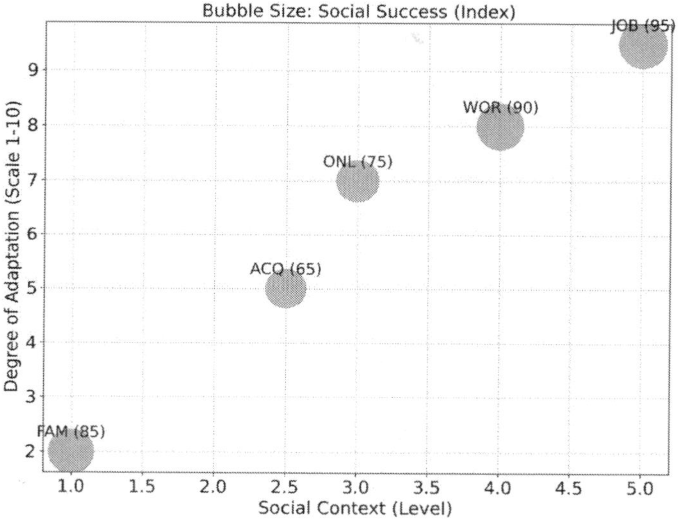

Blasengröße: Social Success (Index)

ACQ: Acquaintances and Hobby

FAM: Family and Close Friends

JOB: Job Interview

ONL: Online Social Media

WOR: Workplace and Colleagues

The chart illustrates that the degree to which individuals adapt their self-presentation (impression management) varies significantly with the social context. In private contexts with family and friends, a low level of adaptation is associated with high social success, as authenticity is valued. As the context becomes more public and formal, such as in the workplace or a job interview, a much higher degree of conscious adaptation is required to achieve desired outcomes like career advancement or a job offer. The size of the bubbles suggests that social success is greatest when the level of adaptation is appropriate for the specific context. An imbalance, such as being overly performative with close friends or too casual in a formal setting, would likely lead to less successful social outcomes. These data points are estimates designed to illustrate these fundamental principles of impression management.

1. 3 Cognitive Dissonance and Attitude Change

Contradictions between beliefs and actions create an inner tension – cognitive dissonance. This state motivates individuals to adjust their attitudes in order to justify their behavior and restore inner balance. This fundamental process continuously shapes self-image and determines whether advice is accepted or rejected. However, this mechanism operates in two directions: it can be used for self-persuasion but can also be abused for manipulation. Understanding this psychological dynamic is crucial for consciously shaping one's own opinion and effectively protecting oneself from external influence. This chapter lays the foundation for the active management of one's social self.

> *The resolution of cognitive dissonance follows the principle of least mental resistance: either one's malleable attitude is adjusted to an irreversible behavior, or external information is devalued to protect a stable conviction.*

> *Two souls, alas! dwell in my breast.*

Johann Wolfgang von Goethe

Faust, Part 1 (1808)
Outside the Gate of the Town

Goethe's famous line, 'Two souls alas! dwell in my breast,' is a powerful metaphor for the internal conflict that lies at the heart of cognitive dissonance. This psychological state arises from holding contradictory beliefs, attitudes, or behaviors simultaneously. The feeling of being torn between two 'souls'—one representing a certain belief and the other a conflicting action—is the very tension that motivates individuals to change their attitudes to restore internal consistency.

1.3.1 Recognizing and Reducing Internal Contradictions

Internal contradictions typically manifest as a vague feeling of discomfort, inner tension, or even guilt. This state is described in social psychology as cognitive dissonance. The drive to reduce this dissonance is fundamentally an attempt to regulate the associated negative emotions. Recognizing this emotional state is the first step in identifying the underlying conflict between beliefs, values, and actions. Once the unpleasant feeling is understood as a signal of an internal contradiction, targeted strategies can be applied to restore inner balance. This process of dissonance reduction is a form of emotion regulation, where various mental pathways are taken to alleviate psychological discomfort [s9].

The reduction of dissonance does not follow a rigid schema but is a flexible process that depends on the intensity of the experienced emotions and the circumstances of the situation. People tend to choose the path of least mental resistance. The most common strategies can be categorized into several groups:

- **Changing behavior or attitude:** The most direct method is to align behavior with belief or, conversely, to change the belief to be consistent with the behavior. For instance, someone who wants to reduce their meat consumption but frequently eats meat experiences dissonance. To reduce it, the person could either actually eat less meat (behavior change) or change their attitude towards meat consumption by re-evaluating and downplaying its negative effects (attitude change).

- **Adding new, consonant cognitions:** Another strategy involves not directly resolving the contradiction but overlaying it with new, supportive thoughts. A person who buys an expensive gadget against their belief in frugality might alleviate their discomfort by focusing on the device's durability, high quality, and future time savings. These new thoughts weaken the original conflict without directly altering it.

- **Trivializing the contradiction:** Here, the relevance of the conflict is downplayed. The contradictory elements are dismissed as unimportant or trivial. In the case of environmentally harmful behavior, such as a short car trip for a small errand, the person might resolve the conflict with their environmental consciousness by telling themselves that this small contribution has no impact in the global context.

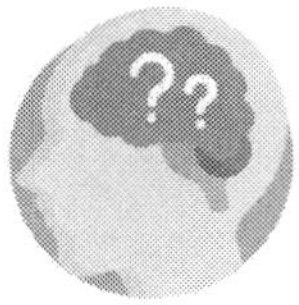

- **Denying personal responsibility:** Dissonance is often reduced by minimizing one's control or responsibility for an action. External circumstances or the influence of others are cited as causes for the dissonant behavior. This relieves the individual of the emotional burden of inconsistency, as the action is perceived as forced or unavoidable.

The choice of strategy is highly individual and context-dependent. A person might initially try to trivialize a contradiction. However, if the negative feeling persists because the contradiction is too strong against fundamental values, they may dynamically switch to another strategy, such as a profound attitude change or seeking justifying information [s9]. A conscious engagement with these mechanisms allows for a better understanding and management of one's reactions. Instead of being unconsciously guided by these automatic processes, one can pause, use the feeling of dissonance as a cue, and consciously decide which solution strategy—such as changing behavior—will ultimately be the most authentic and satisfying.

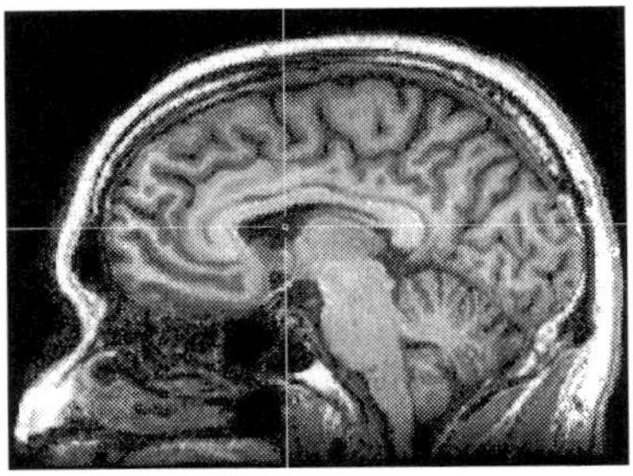

Attitude change [i4]

Good to know

Consonant Cognition

A belief or thought that aligns with a decision made or behavior exhibited. Actively seeking such cognitions serves to justify an action retrospectively.

Dissonance Reduction

The mental process through which a person attempts to resolve the unpleasant state of dissonance. The chosen method often depends on which belief or behavior is easiest to change.

Emotion Regulation

The ability of a person to consciously manage, influence, and adjust their emotional reactions to respond appropriately to a situation or achieve a personal goal.

Inconsistency

The state in which two or more cognitive elements such as thoughts, values, or behaviors of a person are in conflict with each other. This lack of alignment is the actual cause of the feeling of dissonance.

Trivialization

A defense strategy in which the significance or importance of the contradictory behavior or attitude is consciously downplayed. This reduces the emotional weight of the internal conflict.

Effectiveness of Dissonance Reduction Strategies

Estimated effectiveness of various methods for reducing cognitive dissonance

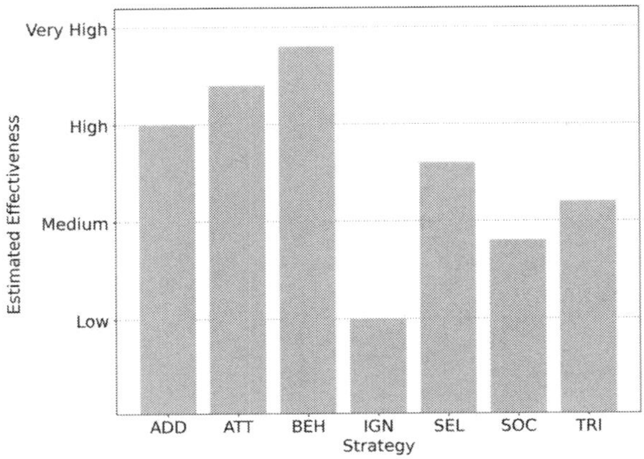

ADD: Adding Consonant Cognitions

ATT: Changing Attitude

BEH: Changing Behavior

IGN: Ignoring/Denying Information

SEL: Self-Affirmation

SOC: Seeking Social Support

TRI: Trivializing the Conflict

The chart illustrates the estimated effectiveness of different psychological strategies for reducing cognitive dissonance. Directly addressing the conflict by changing one's behavior or attitude is shown to be the most effective method. While changing behavior offers the most complete resolution, it is often the most difficult to implement. Changing one's attitude is a powerful and very common alternative. Adding new, consonant cognitions and affirming one's self-worth in other areas are also highly effective indirect methods that reduce the psychological discomfort. Strategies such as trivializing the conflict or seeking social validation offer moderate relief but may not resolve the underlying issue as thoroughly. Ignoring or denying the dissonant information is depicted as the least effective long-term strategy, as it often only provides temporary relief without addressing the core conflict. It is important to emphasize that these values are estimates intended to illustrate the principal mechanisms and relative strengths of the strategies. The actual effectiveness strongly depends on the individual's personality, the specific situation, and the magnitude of the dissonance experienced.

1.3.2 Promoting Self-Conviction Through One's Own Actions

Actions not only influence the external world but also shape the internal landscape of beliefs. One's behavior serves as a powerful source of information about one's own attitudes. Once an action is taken, especially if it was voluntary, individuals strive to evaluate that action retrospectively as meaningful and consistent with their own beliefs. This process of self-conviction through action is a direct consequence of the need to avoid or reduce cognitive dissonance. An action once performed is irreversible; it is often mentally easier to adjust one's attitude to align with the action taken than to live with the internal conflict of having done something that contradicts one's values.

This mechanism has far-reaching implications for the effectiveness of persuasion attempts and advice. When a person receives a persuasive message recommending a certain behavior, the long-term acceptance of that message heavily depends on how the person behaves immediately afterward. If they perform an action that contradicts the recommendation, a dissonance arises between the received message and their own action. To alleviate this mental pressure, the person tends to devalue the original message or justify their own opposing action. The mind's reaction can be compared to a person receiving strict advice to completely refrain from a certain habit, such as consuming fast food. If this person subsequently consumes such a product, an inner conflict arises. Rather than viewing their behavior as a weakness of will, a common reaction is to devalue the advice: "It can't be that bad" or "These strict rules are unrealistic." Through this re-evaluation, the action is justified, dissonance is reduced, and the attitude in favor of fast food consumption is solidified. Consequently, the person may become even more resistant to similar advice in the future, as they have already

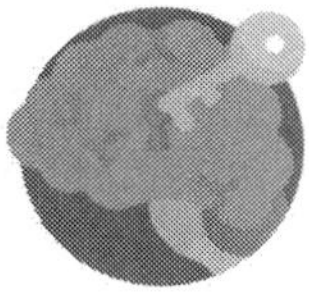

developed a cognitive justification for their behavior [s10].

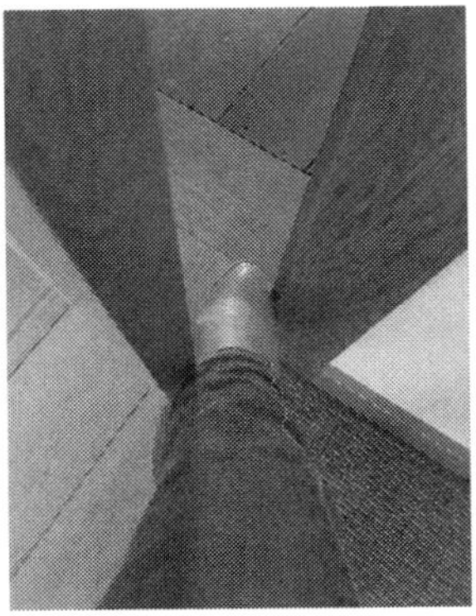

Foot-in-the-door technique [i5]

This principle of self-conviction can be consciously utilized to promote and solidify one's own attitude changes. Instead of merely waiting to be fully immersed in a new belief, the process can be accelerated through targeted actions. Those wishing to develop a more positive attitude towards regular exercise can initiate this through small, concrete actions. It is not about immediately starting an intense training program, but rather about taking an initial, unequivocal action that is consistent with the desired attitude. A short walk in the morning, the conscious decision to take the stairs instead of the elevator, or a ten-minute stretching exercise are such initial actions. Once the action is completed, the mind begins to strengthen the associated attitude to establish consistency. The action provides the evidence: "I am a person who pays attention to their movement." Each subsequent small action in this direction reinforces this new self-perception and gradually builds the corresponding conviction. This approach, often described as the "Foot-in-the-door technique," proactively utilizes dissonance theory: small, voluntary behaviors create minimal dissonance with a previously passive or opposing attitude, which is most easily resolved by adjusting the attitude to align with the new behavior. Thus, the action itself becomes the engine of attitude change.

Good to know

Consistency

Refers to the fundamental human need for one's thoughts, feelings, and actions to be in harmony. A lack of alignment creates an uncomfortable feeling that motivates the adjustment of one's own attitude.

Foot-in-the-door Technique

A persuasion technique in which a person is initially asked for a small, easily granted favor. Agreeing to this request increases the likelihood that the person will later agree to a larger request to align with their previous behavior.

Resistance

Describes a person's psychological resilience to attempts at attitude change. This can be strengthened when arguments have already been developed to defend one's own, divergent action.

Persuasion

Refers to the targeted attempt to influence a person's attitudes, beliefs, or behavior through communication. The effectiveness depends on whether the addressed person mentally processes and accepts the message.

Effort Justification Effect

Shows the positive correlation between the effort invested in an action and the subsequent strength of attitude change.

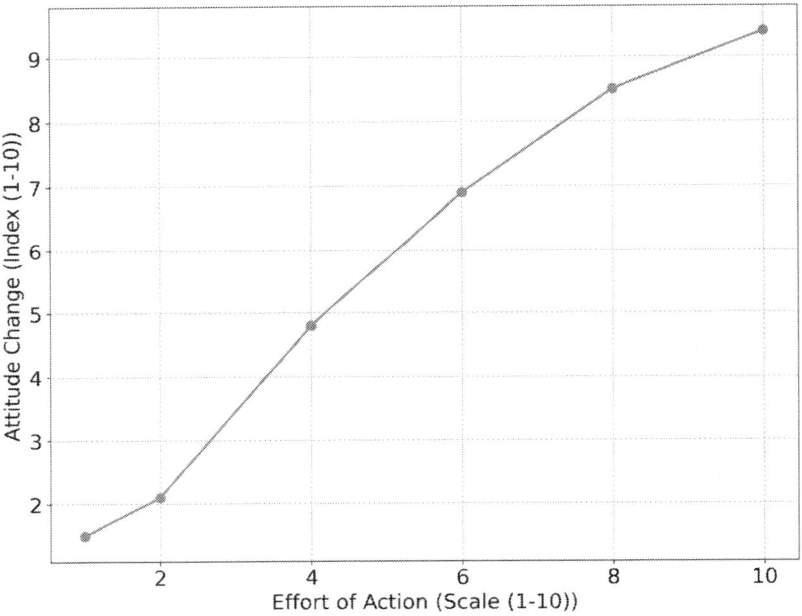

The diagram illustrates a clear positive trend: the greater the effort invested in an action, the more significant the resulting change in attitude. Individuals who expend minimal effort show only a slight shift in their beliefs. However, as the personal investment (e.g., time, difficulty, or resources) increases, the subsequent change in attitude becomes substantially stronger. This pattern reflects the principle of effort justification, a mechanism for resolving cognitive dissonance. To make sense of our significant effort, we subconsciously increase the value we place on the outcome, leading to a more profound and lasting conviction that the action was worthwhile. The presented data are representative estimates intended to visualize this well-established psychological principle.

1.3.3 Strengthening Resilience Against Opinion Manipulation

Resilience to external persuasion attempts is based on the ability to recognize manipulative intentions and actively defend one's own attitudes. While self-persuasion through personal action represents an internal adjustment, protection against external influence requires a conscious engagement with the motives of others. An effective protective mechanism against such influences is the so-called inoculation. This theory posits that individuals become more resistant to strong persuasive messages when they are first exposed to a weakened version of these arguments and are simultaneously informed about the intent to influence [s11]. Through this "cognitive preparation," the mental immune system is activated. The individual is motivated to defend their existing beliefs and begins to actively develop counterarguments. Instead of being caught off guard by a strong message that creates dissonance and suggests an attitude change, the person already possesses an argumentative repertoire to fend off the persuasion attempt.

This principle finds diverse applications in everyday life, especially in the digital realm, where the boundaries between authentic opinion and targeted manipulation often blur. A flood of online comments that presents a uniformly positive or negative opinion about a product, service, or political issue can create a strong opinion landscape. Individuals with little prior experience or uncertainty tend to align their stance with this apparent opinion climate to achieve social conformity and avoid cognitive dissonance. Awareness of the existence of paid reviews or coordinated campaigns acts like the aforementioned inoculation. Someone who is aware of the common practice of purchased product reviews or strategically placed political comments reads these texts with a different mindset. Knowledge of the potential manipulative intent prompts a defensive processing of the information [s11]. Attention shifts from mere content absorption to critical analysis of the source and its possible motives. Instead of questioning their own attitude, the credibility of the external message is downgraded.

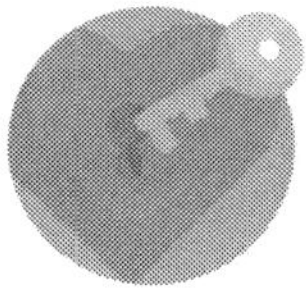

The practical strengthening of resilience therefore involves several steps that build on this mechanism:

- **Creating awareness of manipulation strategies:** The first step is active information about common techniques of opinion influence. Knowing that algorithms create echo chambers or that social media is used for targeted disinformation campaigns changes the perception of the presented content.
- **Actively questioning motives:** Instead of passively consuming information, the question of intent behind a message should become routine. Who benefits if I adopt this opinion? What goal does the person or organization disseminating this information pursue?
- **Developing counterarguments:** When confronted with a persuasive message that contradicts one's beliefs, it is helpful to consciously seek out counterpositions and supporting arguments for one's stance. This process solidifies one's attitude and protects it from erosion by one-sided representations.

Through this cognitive preparation, the automatic dissonance reduction through attitude change is interrupted. The inner conflict created by a persuasive message is no longer primarily resolved by adjusting one's opinion. Instead, dissonance is reduced by classifying the external information as untrustworthy, manipulative, or irrelevant. This ability to critically evaluate the source and its intention leads to a lower identification with the sender of the message and forms the basis for stable and self-determined opinion formation in an information-rich environment.

Good to know

Echo Chamber

A social or informational environment in which existing opinions are reinforced through repeated confirmation and divergent perspectives are excluded. Such environments hinder the correction of misjudgments and can lead to one's own stance being perceived as more universally valid than it actually is.

Disinformation Campaign

The strategic and often coordinated dissemination of false or misleading information with the aim of shaping public opinion, sowing distrust, or destabilizing the attitudes of a target group. Unlike misinformation, this occurs with a conscious intent to deceive.

Identification

The process by which a person adopts the characteristics, values, or attitudes of another person or group as part of their own self. A high identification with the sender of a message increases the likelihood of an attitude change, as adopting the foreign opinion is perceived as a confirmation of one's own belonging.

Inoculation

A procedure in which a person is encouraged to strengthen their own attitude through targeted confrontation with weak counterarguments. Similar to a medical vaccination, this process strengthens defenses against later, stronger attempts at influence by making one's own position conscious and ready to defend.

Factors of Resilience Against Opinion Manipulation

Estimated contribution of different psychological factors to resilience against manipulation.

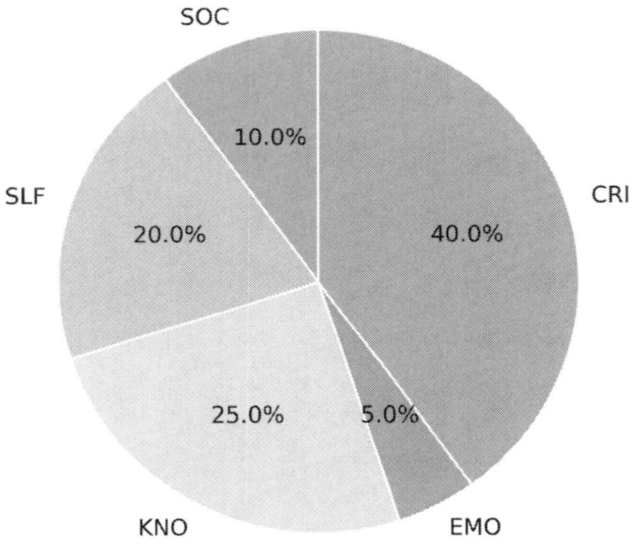

CRI: Critical Thinking and Media Literacy
EMO: Emotional Regulation
KNO: Prior Knowledge and Conviction
SLF: Self-Concept and Self-Esteem
SOC: Social Support

The chart illustrates the estimated relative importance of various psychological factors in building resilience against opinion manipulation. It suggests that cognitive abilities, such as critical thinking and media literacy, are the most significant component, accounting for the largest portion of an individual's defense. Strong prior knowledge and conviction on a topic also form a major line of defense against attitude change. Personal factors like high self-esteem and a stable self-concept act as a crucial internal buffer. Furthermore, a supportive social network and the ability to regulate emotional responses are shown to be important, albeit smaller, contributors. These figures are principled estimates intended to represent the interplay and general weighting of these mechanisms, rather than precise empirical data from a single study.

Concrete Advice

- Consciously play the 'Devil's Advocate' for one of your deep convictions by formulating the three strongest counterarguments in writing to train your mental flexibility.
- Use your future ideal self as a guide by asking yourself in moments of doubt which action brings you one step closer to that ideal image.
- Increase your commitment to a new goal by making a conscious, symbolic effort, such as purchasing a high-quality specialized book, thereby justifying the effort to yourself.
- In a thought experiment or a harmless discussion, temporarily defend the opinion you actually reject to break the rigidity of your own position.
- Give a name to the inner voice that justifies your contradictory behavior to distance yourself from it and view its arguments as external suggestions rather than inner truths.
- Cement a decision you have made by immediately creating a list of all the advantages of your choice and consciously forbidding yourself to think about the discarded alternative for 48 hours.
- Physically locate the feeling of inner contradiction—such as pressure in your stomach—and use this sensation as a trained early warning system for inconsistent behavior.
- Keep a 'Justification Log' to uncover the recurring excuses you use to excuse behavior that actually contradicts your true values.
- Shape your environment so that behavior aligned with your values becomes the path of least resistance, for example, by laying out your sports clothes the night before.

Review - 1. The Social Self: Perception and Influence of One's Own Person

The journey towards understanding one's own social self often begins with an uncomfortable realization: our perception of ourselves is rarely an objective judgment, but rather the result of constant, mostly unconscious comparison processes. Especially in a digitally connected world, where idealized life designs are ubiquitous, this automatism can lead to a downward spiral of self-doubt. However, the key to a more stable and simultaneously realistic self-view lies not in suppressing these comparisons, but in consciously managing them and expanding one's toolkit for self-reflection. Instead of measuring oneself solely against others, one can deliberately shift the focus. Ask yourself not only, "Am I as successful as my peers?" but rather, "What concrete progress have I made in the past year?" (temporal comparison) or "In which areas of my life do my actual strengths lie, even if I still have room for development in others?" (dimensional comparison). A practical exercise for this is personal inventory: take conscious time, perhaps once a month, to evaluate the various pillars of your identity—career, relationships, hobbies, personal development—separately and to acknowledge the successes and resources in each area. The greatest hurdle here is the initial confrontation with one's own shortcomings, but this honest assessment creates the foundation for genuine, self-directed growth that is independent of external validation.

Building on this sharpened self-image, the question arises of how we can authentically carry this into the social world without bending ourselves or remaining stuck in a rigid role. The often-perceived contradiction between authenticity and strategic self-presentation can be understood as a conscious balancing act. It is not about creating a false persona, but about selecting from the diversity of one's own facets those that are purposeful and appropriate in a specific context. Establish a brief "Context-Goal-Authenticity-Check" for yourself before entering important social situations: What is the framework (e.g., formal meeting, casual team event)? What is my goal (e.g., conveying competence, building trust)? And how can I achieve this goal in a way that aligns with my core values? For instance, an introverted leader does not need to mimic a loud, extroverted style to be perceived as competent. They can authentically fulfill their role by impressing through excellent preparation, active listening, and clear, thoughtful communication. The challenge lies in understanding this flexibility not as a lack of integrity, but as an expression of social intelligence that enables effective connection with different people without losing oneself.

One's own actions are the most powerful engine for shaping our beliefs. Often, we wait to be convinced of a stance before we act. However, social psychology shows us that it is often more effective to do the opposite: act your way into your new belief. For example, if you want to work on your inner attitude to be more open towards others, do not wait for the feeling of openness. Instead, take a small, concrete action that corresponds to this attitude. The "method of the smallest effective step" proves particularly powerful here. Resolve to ask a single person an open question at the next opportunity. Once this action is taken, your mind begins to justify this act and adjust your self-perception: "I am a person who seeks contact." This process of self-persuasion also protects against external manipulation. Those who understand the mechanisms of their own dissonance reduction simultaneously develop a finer sensitivity to external attempts to create internal contradictions in order to influence opinions. The most challenging task in this approach is to overcome the initial resistance and to avoid the easier path of rationalizing excuses. Yet every small, conscious step strengthens the "muscle" of self-efficacy and solidifies the foundation for a stable, internally guided identity.

Ultimately, engaging with the social self is not a project with a fixed endpoint, but a lifelong, dynamic process. It is not about constructing a perfect, unchanging self, but about mastering the ability to consciously direct one's perception, authentically adapt one's presence to contexts, and use internal contradictions as impulses for growth. You transition from being a passive object of social evaluations to an active architect of your own social experiences. It is the path to an authentic way of life, where the social self is no longer a source of uncertainty, but an expression of strength, awareness, and genuine connection.

2. Social Influence: Persuasion Strategies and Conformity Pressure

Why do people agree to decisions they would never have made on their own? Daily, we are influenced by others – sometimes consciously and strategically, sometimes through the subtle pressure of the group or the power of authority figures. These processes follow psychological laws that often shape our behavior more than rational considerations. Whether in advertising, at the workplace, or within our circle of friends: social influence is omnipresent and often operates below the threshold of consciousness. Understanding the mechanisms that lead us to yield, agree, or obey provides a fascinating insight into the power of interpersonal dynamics.

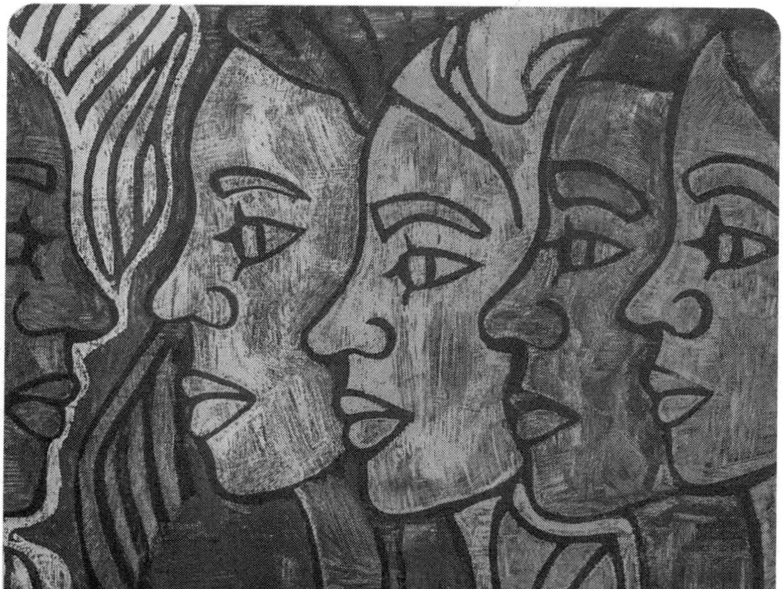

Landmarks of Social Influence

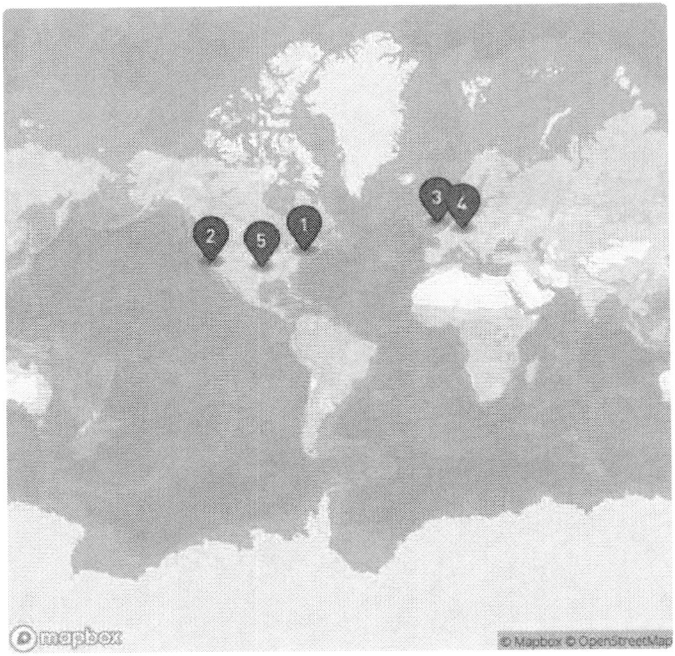

A map of landmark experiments and locations that shaped our understanding of social conformity and obedience to authority.

1 **Yale University, New Haven, USA**

Site of Stanley Milgram's infamous obedience experiments in 1961. In the wake of the Holocaust, Milgram wanted to test the 'just following orders' defense. Participants, assigned as 'teachers', were instructed by an authority figure to deliver what they believed were increasingly painful electric shocks to a 'learner'. A staggering 65% of participants administered the final, seemingly lethal, 450-volt shock, demonstrating the powerful and unsettling human tendency to obey authority, even against their own conscience.

2 **Stanford University, Palo Alto, USA**

Location of Philip Zimbardo's 1971 Stanford Prison Experiment. Healthy male students were randomly assigned to be 'prisoners' or 'guards' in a simulated prison. The study, planned for two weeks, was terminated after only six days. The 'guards' quickly became authoritarian and abusive, while the 'prisoners' became passive and distressed. The experiment demonstrated how readily people conform to prescribed social roles and situational pressures, showing that the 'power of the situation' can often override individual personality.

3 **University of Bristol, Bristol, UK**

Here, Henri Tajfel and colleagues developed the Minimal Group Paradigm in the 1970s. They demonstrated that even when groups are formed on the most trivial and arbitrary criteria (e.g., preference for a painter), people will favor their own group (in-group) over the other (out-group). This research formed the basis of Social Identity Theory, showing that a core part of our identity comes from group membership, which drives in-group conformity and can be a root cause of prejudice and discrimination.

4 **Nuremberg Palace of Justice, Germany**

This location is not an experiment, but the historical catalyst for obedience research. After WWII, the Nuremberg Trials were held here to prosecute Nazi war criminals. Many defendants claimed they were 'just following orders'. This 'Nuremberg Defense' directly inspired Stanley Milgram's experiments at Yale, as he sought to scientifically investigate whether ordinary people would commit immoral acts under the direction of an authority figure.

5 **Robbers Cave State Park, Oklahoma, USA**
The setting for Muzafer Sherif's 1954 'Robbers Cave' field experiment. Two groups of 11-year-old boys, the 'Eagles' and the 'Rattlers', were brought to a summer camp. Sherif first fostered strong in-group identity and then created intergroup conflict through competition. This led to intense hostility. The key finding was that the conflict was only resolved when the groups were forced to cooperate on 'superordinate goals'—tasks that required them to work together. It highlighted how group norms, conformity, and conflict are highly dependent on the situation.

2. 1 Mechanisms of Targeted Persuasion

Targeted persuasion requires more than sound arguments. The success of a message depends on whether it encounters an analytically thinking or a superficially judging recipient. People utilize different cognitive pathways depending on their motivation and ability: sometimes they critically examine facts, while at other times they rely on mental shortcuts such as sympathy for the speaker or the behavior of the majority. This chapter reveals the psychological principles underlying these processes. It demonstrates how universal heuristics like reciprocity, social proof, and authority shape attitudes and actions, often without the recipient's conscious deliberation. Mastering these mechanisms is key to precisely steering messages and achieving their intended effect.

> *Successful persuasion depends less on the strength of the argument than on the targeted use of psychological levers that unconsciously guide our decisions.*

> *It is simplicity that makes the uneducated more effective than the educated when addressing popular audiences.*

Aristotle

Rhetoric
Book II, 1395b.27

Aristotle, in his foundational work on rhetoric, identifies a key principle of persuasion that remains central to social psychology. The effectiveness of a message often depends less on its intellectual complexity and more on its clarity and relatability to the audience. This insight explains why simple, emotionally resonant arguments can be more persuasive in mass communication than detailed, fact-based ones, a mechanism often exploited in advertising and political campaigns.

2.1.1 Application of Central and Peripheral Persuasion Routes

The targeted application of persuasion routes depends on the motivation and ability of the recipient to process a message. The Elaboration Likelihood Model describes two fundamental pathways through which people receive information and change their attitudes: the central and the peripheral route. The choice of the appropriate route determines the effectiveness of a message.

The central route of persuasion requires a high cognitive effort from the audience. Individuals who take this path are motivated to engage deeply with a topic and possess the necessary time and prior knowledge to critically evaluate arguments. Persuasion occurs here through the quality and logic of the presented facts. An attitude formed through this route is generally stable, long-lasting, and resistant to counterarguments. For this reason, the central route is suitable for messages intended to bring about a well-founded and lasting change in attitude, such as in complex purchasing decisions or political positioning. Processing through this route demonstrably requires significant cognitive resources, which is reflected in increased brain activity during attention-demanding tasks [s12]. Therefore, anyone wishing to address an audience that already has an interest in the topic and is willing to reflect should rely on sound, well-structured, and comprehensible arguments. The sheer quantity of arguments is less decisive than their substantive content.

In contrast, the peripheral route is based on superficial processing of information. It is taken when the audience is unmotivated, distracted, or cognitively overloaded. Instead of engaging with the content of a message, people rely on heuristic cues. Such cues are easily processed mental shortcuts that allow for quick, albeit often less informed, judgments. These include the perceived credibility or attractiveness of the communicator, the number of arguments presented (regardless of their quality), positive or negative moods, or the reactions of others.

Especially in crisis situations or when there is a high density of information, as prevalent in digital media, people tend to prefer receiving information through the peripheral route [s13]. The sheer volume of stimuli makes a deeper analysis of each individual message impossible. In such environments, peripheral cues can be extremely effective. A social media campaign promoting protective measures can increase the dissemination of information if it conveys positive emotions such as hope or a sense of community, rather than relying solely on the sober presentation of statistics [s13]. Negative emotions can also, contextually, promote the spread of content. Attention studies show that even simple text-based peripheral cues are sufficient to enhance early attention engagement and pique the recipient's interest [s12]. However, attitudes formed through this route are often less stable and more susceptible to later attempts at influence.

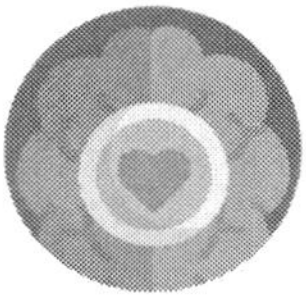

For an effective persuasion strategy, the situational combination of both routes is beneficial. The strategic application depends on the goal and the state of the audience.

- To capture the attention of a broad, possibly disinterested audience, peripheral cues are initially suitable. An engaging speaker, an emotionally charged image, or a surprising slogan can serve as "door openers" to spark interest for deeper engagement.
- Once initial attention is secured, central arguments can be provided for that part of the audience that now shows motivation for further engagement. This can transform superficial agreement into a solid conviction.

The conscious management of persuasion routes allows for precise alignment of communication measures with the respective target group and context. Success lies not in favoring a single route, but in understanding when logical arguments resonate and when emotional or heuristic cues pave the way for a message.

Good to know

Central Route

A processing path chosen primarily when a topic is of high personal significance to an individual. Attitudes formed through this route predict a person's future behavior more reliably.

Cognitive Resource

Refers to the limited mental capacity available for demanding thought processes. Since this capacity is limited, people cannot process all information deeply and often resort to simplifications.

Elaboration Likelihood Model

A model developed by psychologists Richard E. Petty and John T. Cacioppo that explains under what conditions people think about the arguments of a message. The likelihood of cognitive engagement determines the path of attitude change.

Heuristic Cue

Mental shortcuts that enable quick judgment without in-depth analysis. Examples include the assumption that a longer message has more substance or that an expert's opinion is always correct.

Peripheral Route

A processing path where attitudes are shaped by associating a message with simple positive or negative cues. For example, a brand presented repeatedly with pleasant music may seem more likable without any thought about the product itself.

Effectiveness of Persuasion Routes

Comparison of Central vs. Peripheral Route Impact on Attitude and Behavior

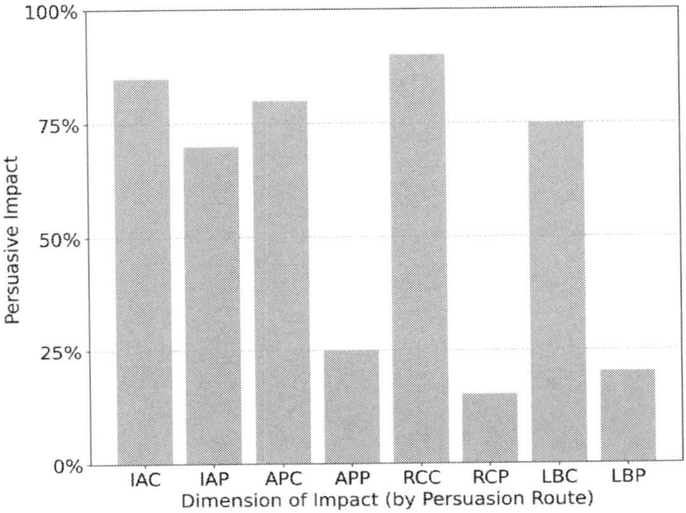

APC: Attitude Persistence (Central)
APP: Attitude Persistence (Peripheral)
IAC: Immediate Attitude Change (Central)
IAP: Immediate Attitude Change (Peripheral)
LBC: Link to Behavior (Central)
LBP: Link to Behavior (Peripheral)
RCC: Resistance to Countering (Central)
RCP: Resistance to Countering (Peripheral)

The chart illustrates the distinct effects of the two primary routes of persuasion. While both central and peripheral routes can achieve significant immediate attitude change, the central route, which involves deep cognitive processing of the message, leads to outcomes that are substantially more stable and robust. Attitudes formed via the central route show much greater persistence over time, are more resistant to subsequent counter-arguments, and are more reliable in predicting actual behavior. In contrast, the peripheral route, relying on superficial cues, results in more transient and fragile attitude changes with a weaker link to behavior. Please note: The values presented are illustrative estimates designed to represent the fundamental principles of the Elaboration Likelihood Model, not data from a single specific study.

2.1.2 The Effective Use of Reciprocity and Social Proof

Reciprocity and social proof are two deeply rooted social heuristics that predictably influence human behavior. They are not based on the logical strength of arguments but on automated responses that arise from societal norms. Their application allows for a subtle and effective form of persuasion.

The principle of reciprocity describes the universal human tendency to reciprocate a received benefit with a return favor. This norm of "give and take" is embedded in all cultures and creates a sense of obligation. When a person receives an unsolicited gift, a favor, or a concession, a psychological discomfort arises that can only be resolved by reciprocation. This need to "repay a debt" is often so strong that the return favor can exceed the value of the original gift. To leverage this mechanism, a communicator can precede a request with a positive action. For instance, distributing free product samples in a supermarket can increase the likelihood of purchase, not only because the product tastes good but because a small social obligation has been established.

An advanced application of this rule is the "Door-in-the-Face Technique" (Door-in-the-Face Technique). Here, an exaggerated, unrealistic demand is initially made, which the counterpart is likely to reject. Immediately afterward, a second, significantly smaller request is presented – the actual target request. The withdrawal of the first demand is perceived by the recipient as a concession or concession. This "gift" of yielding triggers the reciprocity impulse to also make a concession by agreeing to the smaller request. A requester who initially asks for a large monthly donation and then shifts to a much smaller one-time contribution utilizes this effect. The perceived gesture of concession generates an impulse in the counterpart to also yield and agree to the smaller request. The effectiveness depends on the second request following directly after the first and being perceived as part of the same negotiation.

Closely related to these social automatons is the principle of social proof. It states that individuals align their behavior with that of others. Particularly in situations of uncertainty, where it is unclear what behavior is appropriate or correct, the actions of the majority serve as a guide and mental shortcut. When many people make a particular choice, it is assumed that this choice is good or correct. This principle explains the effectiveness of customer reviews, bestseller lists, or the indication of user numbers. The information "millions of satisfied customers" suggests that a purchase cannot be a wrong decision.

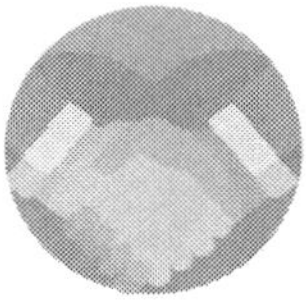

The strength of social proof increases under two conditions:
- **Uncertainty:** The less a person knows about a situation or the more ambiguous the circumstances are, the more they rely on the actions of others.
- **Similarity:** The actions of individuals who are similar to us (in age, background, interests) have a greater influence on our decisions. Testimonials from peers are therefore more persuasive than those from experts who are perceived as dissimilar.

To strategically employ social proof, positive behaviors of a relevant reference group can be made visible. For example, the information on a booking platform that a property has already been viewed multiple times by other users for the same period can accelerate one's own decision. The actions of the majority serve as validation and reduce the perceived uncertainty in the choice. However, it should be noted that this mechanism can also have negative consequences, such as in the case of pluralistic ignorance, where in an emergency situation no one intervenes because everyone is following the passive behavior of others. A conscious application, therefore, focuses on promoting desired behavior by presenting a positive social norm.

Good to know

Door-in-the-Face Technique

A persuasion tactic based on an apparent compromise. Its effectiveness crucially depends on the first, large request being rejected, but not so extreme that it makes the requester appear unserious. The second, smaller request must be perceived as a reasonable and sincere correction of the first demand.

Pluralistic Ignorance

A group state in which the majority of members privately reject a norm or belief but mistakenly assume that most others accept it. Each individual adjusts their public behavior to this perceived norm, thereby confirming the false assumption for everyone.

Social Proof

A psychological phenomenon where a person views the actions of a large group as evidence of the correct behavior. This often occurs unconsciously and serves as a mental shortcut to simplify complex decisions. The underlying assumption is that the majority is likely not wrong, which is particularly exploited during the introduction of new products or ideas.

Effectiveness of Persuasion Techniques

A comparison of the success rate of different psychological persuasion techniques.

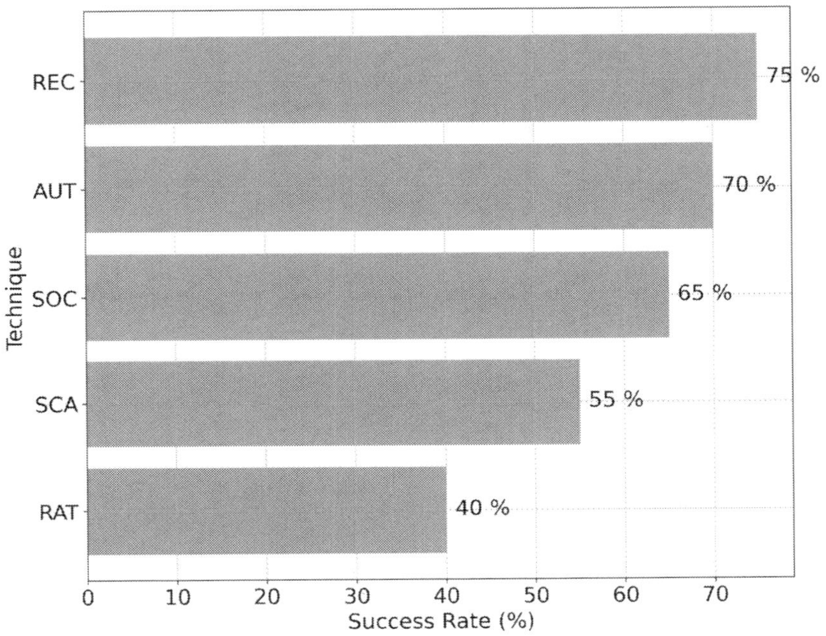

AUT: Authority

REC: Reciprocity

SOC: Social Proof

RAT: Rational Argument

SCA: Scarcity

The chart compares the estimated effectiveness of several key persuasion techniques. Techniques such as Reciprocity and Authority, which appeal to deep-seated psychological triggers, show a significantly higher success rate than a purely rational argument. Social Proof also proves to be a very effective method, capitalizing on the human tendency to follow the actions of others. It is important to note that these values are estimates intended to illustrate the general principles of their effectiveness. In practice, the success of any technique can vary greatly depending on the context, audience, and execution. The key takeaway is that leveraging psychological principles is often more persuasive than relying on logic alone.

2.1.3 The Use of Liking and Authority in Argumentation

People tend to comply more with requests from individuals they like. This phenomenon, known as the principle of liking, is based on an emotional connection rather than a rational evaluation of arguments. Affection for a communicator can be triggered and deliberately enhanced by various factors to increase the likelihood of agreement. One such factor is physical attractiveness, which triggers the halo effect: Attractive individuals are unconsciously attributed additional positive traits such as honesty, intelligence, and competence. Their arguments thus carry more weight, even if they are not substantively superior.

Another effective factor is similarity. We feel affinity for people who share our opinions, backgrounds, lifestyles, or even external characteristics such as clothing. Establishing such common ground creates a basis of trust and connection. A salesperson who casually mentions a shared hobby or regional background during a conversation with a customer builds a personal bridge. This connection makes the other party more receptive to suggestions, as the interaction is perceived less as a mere sales pitch and more as an exchange between like-minded individuals. Genuine compliments and praise also enhance liking, as does collaboration on a common goal. People with whom we successfully cooperate are evaluated more positively and are more likely to be followed in other matters. Therefore, to create a positive relationship as a foundation for persuasion, it is useful to actively seek out and address authentic commonalities or to establish a cooperative atmosphere before making the actual request.

In addition to personal affection, the perceived authority of a person is another strong factor in persuasion. From early childhood, individuals learn to comply with the instructions of authority figures such as parents, teachers, and experts. This behavior serves as a useful mental shortcut, relieving us from having to analyze every situation independently in detail. We rely on experts to possess sound knowledge and adopt their judgments. This tendency is so deeply ingrained that often mere symbols of authority are sufficient to trigger automatic compliance.

These symbols can be categorized into three groups:
- **Titles:** A "Dr." or "Professor" before a name immediately lends more weight to a statement, regardless of its content.

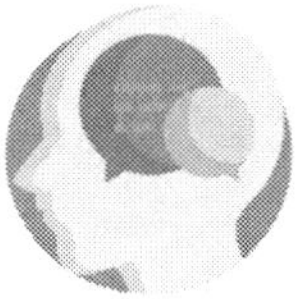

- **Clothing:** Uniforms or specific professional attire, such as a doctor's coat or a business suit, signal a certain status and expertise. An actor in a lab coat promoting a medical product exploits this effect by suggesting competence without possessing it.
- **External Accessories:** Status symbols such as expensive cars, luxurious offices, or high-quality watches can also be perceived as evidence of success and thus of competence and authority.

Appealing to authority is a common persuasion technique. Instead of detailing the advantages of a product, advertisers refer to the judgment of experts ("recommended by dentists"). The persuasive power here does not depend on the argument itself but on the credibility of the cited source. To be perceived as an authority, one does not necessarily have to rely on titles or status symbols. One's expertise can be subtly and often more effectively supported by explaining complex issues in an understandable manner or by presenting relevant experiences and successes from the past. This demonstration of expertise creates a legitimate basis for authority that goes beyond mere symbols and allows for a more substantiated form of persuasion. Both liking and authority thus primarily operate through the peripheral route of information processing, bypassing critical engagement with the actual content of a message.

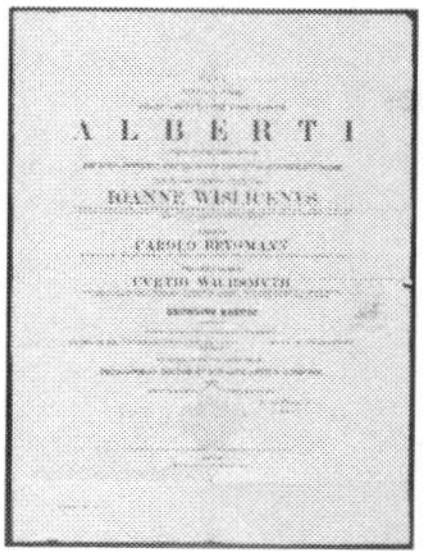

Doctorate [i6]

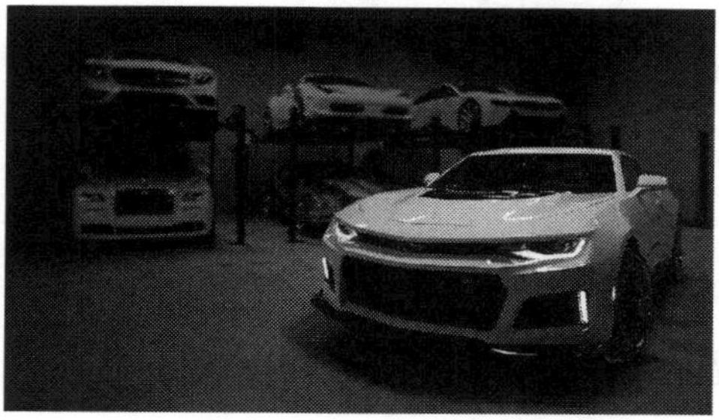

luxury car [i7]

Good to know

Authority

Refers to the influence attributed to a person based on their perceived position, knowledge, or status. Their persuasive power is particularly high when deemed legitimate and appropriate for the respective matter.

Communicator

Refers to the source or sender of a persuasive message. The impact of the communicator depends not only on likability or authority but significantly on their perceived credibility, which consists of their competence and trustworthiness.

Halo Effect

A cognitive bias in which a single, prominent trait of a person, such as physical attractiveness, positively colors the overall perception of that person. The opposite of this phenomenon, where a negative trait leads to a general devaluation, is referred to as the horn effect.

Principle of Liking

A principle of persuasion whose effectiveness is based on the human need for social bonds. A rejection of a request from a likable person is often avoided, as it can be unconsciously perceived as a threat to the social relationship.

Die Macht der Überzeugung

Überzeugungserfolg in Bezug auf die wahrgenommene Sympathie und Autorität des Kommunikators.

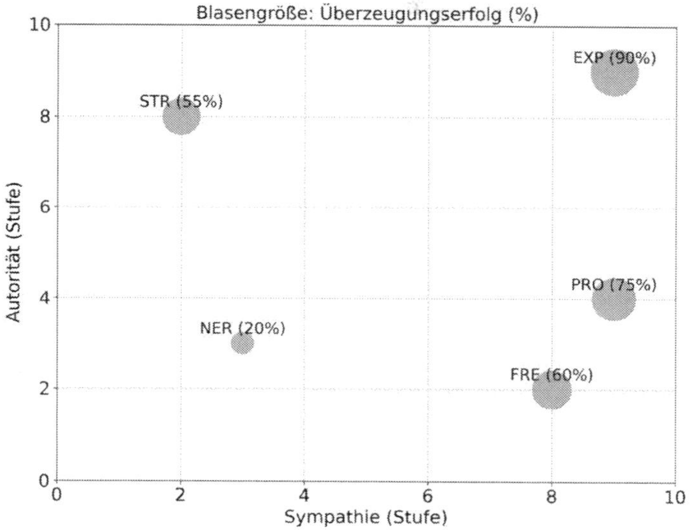

Blasengröße: Überzeugungserfolg (%)

EXP: Vertrauenswürdiger Experte

FRE: Guter Freund

NER: Nerviger Verkäufer

PRO: Promi-Endorser

STR: Strenger Offizier

Diese Daten sind Schätzungen, die grundlegende Prinzipien der Sozialpsychologie veranschaulichen sollen. Die Grafik zeigt, dass Überzeugung am effektivsten ist, wenn hohe Sympathie mit hoher Autorität kombiniert wird, wie beim 'Vertrauenswürdigen Experten'. Beide Faktoren sind jedoch auch für sich genommen wirkungsvoll. Der 'Gute Freund' und der 'Promi-Endorser' zeigen, dass hohe Sympathie sehr überzeugend sein kann, selbst bei geringerer Fachautorität. Umgekehrt kann ein 'Strenger Offizier' mit hoher Autorität trotz geringer Sympathie ebenfalls einen erheblichen Überzeugungserfolg erzielen. Der 'Nervige Verkäufer', dem es sowohl an Sympathie als auch an Autorität mangelt, ist erwartungsgemäß am wenigsten effektiv. Dies verdeutlicht, dass Überzeugung ein komplexes Zusammenspiel sozialer Faktoren ist und kein einfacher, eindimensionaler Prozess.

Concrete Advice

- Create a 'mental workshop' where you present not finished solutions to your counterpart, but the building blocks of an argument, allowing them to feel as though they have arrived at the conclusion themselves.
- Deliberately evoke a sense of personal responsibility or curiosity before laying out the factual arguments to enhance motivation for a deeper analysis.
- Utilize the principle of 'future validity' by referring not to the broad masses, but to a small, yet growing group of pioneers whose behavior is considered exemplary.
- Borrow authority not only through quotes but by clearly explaining the thought process of an expert, thereby acquiring their analytical competence.
- Attribute a positive quality to your counterpart, for example, 'As someone who always weighs things fairly...', before making a request that specifically requires that quality.
- Articulate your core message in a simple, rhythmic sentence, as the ease of cognitive processing is unconsciously equated with correctness.
- Establish a desired norm by demonstrating which behavior a group avoids, to which your counterpart clearly does not want to belong.
- Anchor the value of your proposal by presenting it immediately after mentioning a significantly more costly or less attractive alternative.
- Grant an exclusive knowledge advantage by sharing valuable information that is not widely known, thereby creating a reciprocal inclination towards agreement.

2. 2 Dealing with Group Pressure and Conformity

The human need for belonging often conflicts with the maintenance of personal beliefs. Conformity ensures social acceptance but carries the risk of relinquishing one's own values and judgments. This tension presents individuals with the daily challenge of preserving their autonomy without risking social rejection. At the same time, the belief in the correctness of the majority opinion often leads to uncritical imitation. This pressure to conform not only jeopardizes personal judgment but can also lead entire groups to make erroneous decisions. This chapter imparts the essential skills to navigate this tension with confidence.

True resistance to group pressure does not sabotage the group, but rather protects it from the errors of unanimity.

Morality is herd instinct in the individual.

Friedrich Nietzsche

The Joyful Wisdom (1882)
Sec. 116

Nietzsche's provocative statement cuts to the core of conformity. He suggests that what we often perceive as personal, objective morality is, in fact, an internalized expression of group norms and the desire to belong—the 'herd instinct'. This reflects the psychological understanding of conformity, where individuals adopt the attitudes and behaviors of a group to gain acceptance and avoid social exclusion, often without conscious awareness of the group's influence.

2.2.1 Resistance to Normative Social Influence

Normative social influence refers to the effort of individuals to conform to the expectations of a group in order to gain social acceptance and avoid rejection. Resistance to this conformity pressure is a process based on a conscious decision to prioritize one's own autonomy over immediate social belonging. This resistance is not a static trait but a skill that depends on situational and personal factors. A central mechanism of resistance is the awareness of the ongoing group process. Individuals who recognize that they are being pressured to adopt a norm that does not align with their own values can mentally isolate this influence and evaluate it more rationally.

Autonomy [i8]

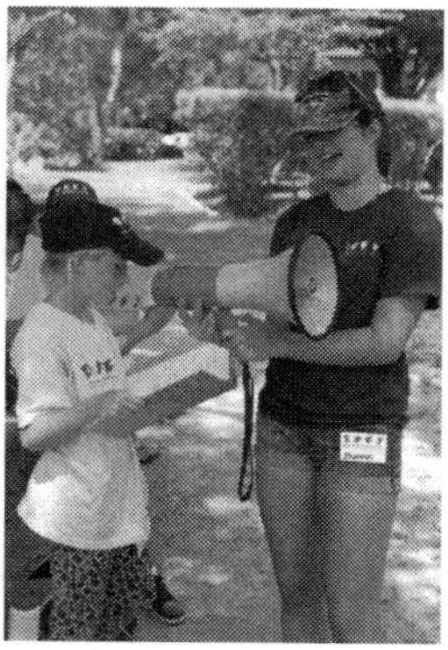

Conformity pressure [i9]

The ability to withstand normative influence develops over the course of life. Research shows that resistance to peer influence particularly increases linearly during adolescence, between the ages of 14 and 18 [s14]. This development correlates with the progressive formation of one's identity and the growing capacity for critical reflection. With a solidified self-image, dependence on external validation from the group decreases, facilitating nonconformity.

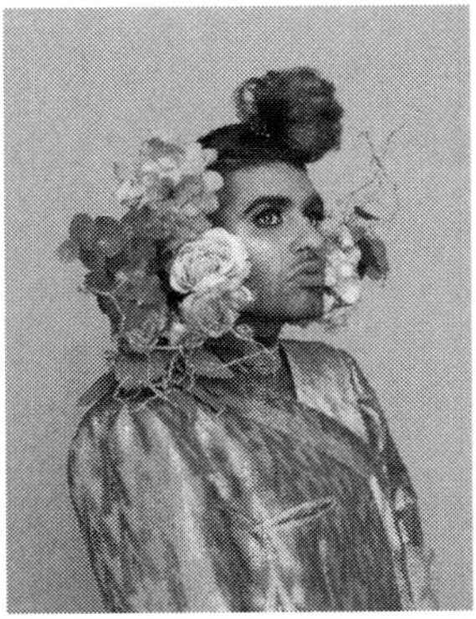

nonconformity [i10]

A very effective strategy for dealing with group pressure is seeking allies. The mere presence of a single other person who also deviates from the group norm drastically reduces conformity pressure. This ally does not even need to share the same dissenting opinion; the fact that the group's unanimity is broken signals that deviant behavior is a legitimate option. This validates one's own position and distributes the social burden of nonconformity across multiple shoulders.

Another factor is the establishment of so-called idiosyncrasy credits. This describes a social "credit" that a person earns through previous conformity and positive contributions to the group. Those who have proven themselves to be loyal and valuable members over time are more likely to be granted occasional deviant behavior without immediate social exclusion. They have "earned" the right to occasionally swim against the tide. Consciously building and strategically using this credit can lower the social cost of resistance in situations where deviation from the norm is personally warranted.

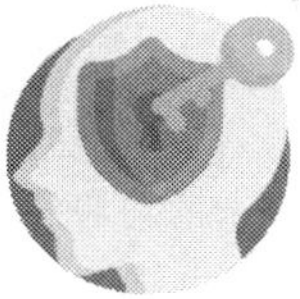

The strength of normative influence is often underestimated, as it operates subtly and appeals to our fundamental need for belonging. For instance, during the COVID-19 pandemic, it was observed that customers' mask-wearing behavior heavily depended on how many other people in the room were already wearing a mask [s15]. A higher number of mask-wearing individuals increased the likelihood that newly arriving customers would also wear one, as a clear social norm became visible. Those wishing to act nonconformingly in such a situation, that is, against the prevailing norm, benefit from conscious self-reflection. A helpful mental exercise is to ask: "Is my current decision based on my own beliefs and assessment of the facts, or primarily on the behavior of the majority?" This brief analysis creates a cognitive distance from the immediate social pressure and allows for more autonomous action. Ultimately, resistance is a trade-off:
- How relevant is the matter to my personal values and beliefs?
- What is the social cost I must pay for my deviation?
- How important is belonging to this particular group to me?

By answering these questions, an informed decision can be made as to whether conformity or resistance is the more appropriate course of action in the given situation.

Good to know

Nonconformity

A behavior that consciously deviates from the established norms or expectations of a group. It can be an expression of individuality or an attempt to challenge an existing norm.

Cognitive Dissonance

A mental state in which a person steps back to observe and evaluate the influence of group dynamics on their own judgment. This allows for more conscious and less reactive decision-making.

Conformity Pressure

The perceived, often unspoken pressure to align one's views or behaviors with the majority of a group. This pressure arises from the expectation that deviation will have negative social consequences.

Idiosyncrasy Credit

An informally granted credit by the group that allows a member to deviate from norms without being punished. This credit is built through previous positive contributions and conformity.

Normative Social Influence

The influence that arises from a person adjusting their actions to those of a group in order to be liked and belong. This process is often emotional and not rational, as the fear of social exclusion serves as a strong motivation.

Strategies for Resisting Group Pressure

Distribution of the effectiveness of different strategies in successfully resisting normative social influence.

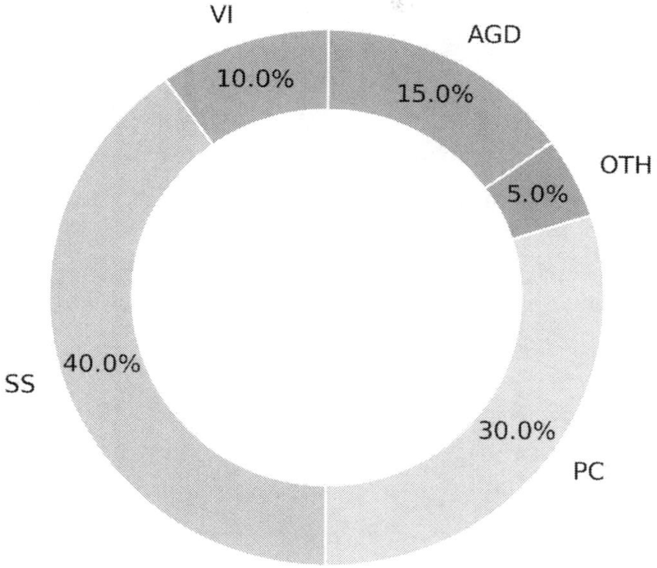

AGD: Awareness of Group Dynamics
PC: Personal Conviction
VI: Valuing Independence
OTH: Other Factors
SS: Social Support / Ally

The data illustrates the relative effectiveness of various strategies in resisting group pressure. The most significant factor for successful resistance is having social support; finding even a single ally who shares your dissenting view can dramatically reduce the pressure to conform. The second most powerful element is a strong, well-founded personal conviction, which serves as an internal anchor against the sway of the majority. Furthermore, a conscious awareness of the psychological dynamics at play and a fundamental personal value placed on independence are also important contributors to resisting conformity. These figures are principled estimates designed to illustrate the key mechanisms of resistance, as the effectiveness of any strategy can vary depending on the specific situation and individual.

2.2.2 Critical Questioning of Majority Opinions

In addition to the desire for social belonging, which underlies the normative influence, there exists a second strong force that governs our behavior in groups: the informational social influence. This describes the tendency to rely on others in ambiguous or uncertain situations because we assume that the actions of the majority reflect a correct interpretation of reality. We use the group as a source of information to arrive at an accurate assessment. This heuristic, or mental shortcut, is often efficient but carries the risk that erroneous assumptions may go unchallenged and lead to poor decisions. Therefore, the critical questioning of majority opinions is a cognitive ability aimed at evaluating the validity of information regardless of the number of its supporters.

A mechanism that undermines critical examination is groupthink. This process occurs particularly in cohesive, strongly bonded groups that are isolated from external opinions and are under pressure to make quick decisions. The pursuit of unanimity then becomes more important than a realistic evaluation of alternatives. Symptoms of groupthink include the illusion of invulnerability, where the group is overly optimistic and ignores risks, as well as collective rationalization, where warning signs and negative feedback are dismissed. Members engage in self-censorship by withholding doubts to avoid disturbing harmony. This creates the illusion of unanimity: silence is mistakenly interpreted as agreement.

Closely related is the phenomenon of pluralistic ignorance. Here, many members of a group privately reject a norm or belief but mistakenly believe that most others accept it. Since no one expresses their dissenting opinion out of fear of the reaction from the supposedly conforming majority, the unpopular norm is maintained publicly. A typical scenario is a complex lecture, after which the instructor asks if there are any questions. Although many listeners have not fully understood the content, no one speaks up, as each assumes they are the only one who has lost track. The collective silence reinforces everyone's false assumption that the group has understood everything. In such situations, a single critical inquiry can break the entire dynamic and reveal that the perceived majority opinion does not actually exist.

Active questioning requires a conscious slowing down of one's thought process. Instead of intuitively following the group opinion, the quality of the arguments should take precedence. The central task is to separate the information from the information source. The validity of a statement does not depend on how many people support it, but on the evidence that supports it. A helpful technique is to mentally adopt the position of an advocatus diaboli. Deliberately ask questions such as: What evidence contradicts the majority's position? What alternative explanations or solutions have been overlooked? Are there conflicts of interest that could influence the group's opinion? Is the opinion formed on a broad information base or only on a single, perhaps biased source?

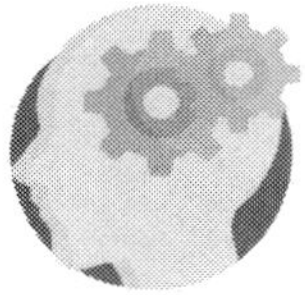

This approach need not be confrontational. In a professional meeting where a team uniformly advocates a particular strategy, questioning can be effectively and constructively framed by focusing on the process and the facts. Instead of directly attacking the conclusion ("I think that's wrong"), it is more productive to ask clarifying and probing questions. This can improve the decision quality for everyone without being perceived as a troublemaker. Concrete formulations can help:
- **Focus on data:** "To fully understand the basis of our decision: Can we take another look at the underlying data that supports this approach?"
- **Request risk analysis:** "That sounds like a promising path. What potential downsides or risks have we identified for this approach, and how do we plan to address them?"
- **Structurally evaluate alternatives:** "To ensure we are absolutely certain we are choosing the best option, could we briefly list the key pros and cons of Alternative B in direct comparison to our favored Plan A?"

Such questions gently guide the group to reflect on their own position, examine assumptions, and uncover blind spots. The goal is not to be right at all costs, but to leverage the collective intelligence of the group to make the most robust and well-founded decision. The ability to question majority opinions thus not only protects one's own autonomy but ultimately serves the success of the group itself.

Good to know

Collective Intelligence

The ability of a group to find better solutions through effective collaboration and the exchange of diverse perspectives than the most capable individual members could alone. Conformity pressure can severely impair this ability.

Collective Rationalization

A common defense mechanism where group members actively seek justifications for their preferred decision while systematically devaluing or ignoring any information that contradicts that decision.

Illusion of Unanimity

A false perception that arises when no dissent is expressed due to self-censorship. It reinforces the group's assumption that they have made the right decision and increases pressure on remaining doubters.

Informational Social Influence

This type of influence often leads to a genuine, internal change of conviction, as the person views the group's information as a reliable indicator of reality and internalizes it.

Pluralistic Ignorance

This phenomenon can explain the inaction of witnesses in emergency situations. Each individual mistakenly interprets the passivity of others as a sign that the situation is not serious.

Group Size and Critical Thinking

This chart illustrates how the likelihood of an individual questioning a majority opinion changes with increasing group size.

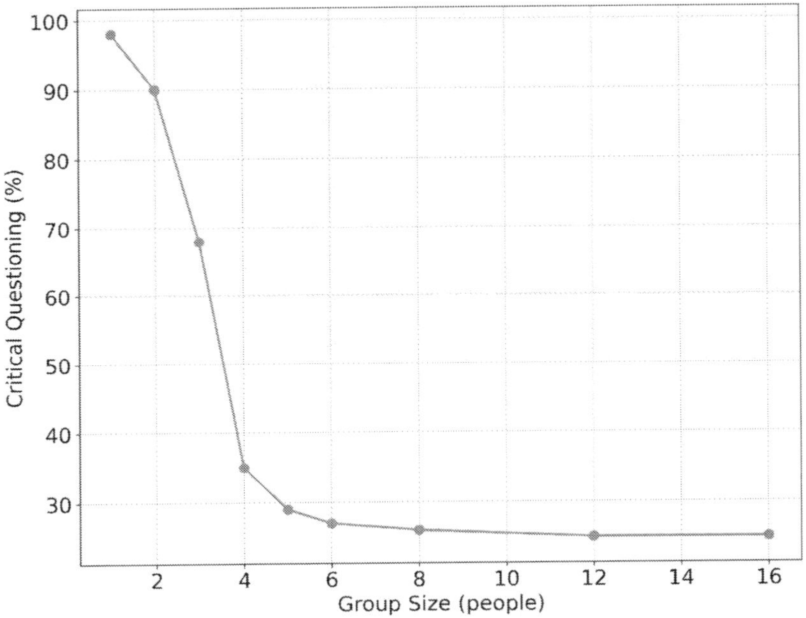

The data illustrates a fundamental principle of social psychology: the pressure to conform increases significantly with the size of the majority group, but only up to a certain point. The probability of an individual critically questioning the group's consensus drops sharply when they are faced with a unanimous majority of three or four people. Beyond this point, adding more members to the majority has a diminishing effect, and the likelihood of dissent stabilizes at a low level. This suggests that the maximum social pressure is reached with a relatively small, but unanimous, group. This is a key insight from classic conformity experiments. Please note that these data are principled estimates designed to visually represent this well-documented psychological effect, rather than being the direct output of a single specific study.

2.2.3 The Role of Allies in Strengthening One's Own Position

Allies provide more than just psychological relief in situations of group pressure. They serve a dual function: they reduce the social cost of deviation while often providing substantive support. The presence of a supporter breaks the monolithic facade of unanimity that can be so intimidating for nonconforming individuals. The mere existence of a second dissenting voice validates one's own position as a legitimate alternative rather than just an isolated, erroneous opinion. The individual's status transforms from a potential troublemaker to a representative of a debatable perspective. This changes the entire social dynamic, as the confrontation shifts from a clash between the group and a deviant to a debate among various viewpoints within the group. The mental pressure arising from the fear of social exclusion is noticeably alleviated, as the risk of rejection is now distributed among several individuals.

Moreover, the benefits of an ally extend far beyond this normative level and encroach upon the realm of informational influence. Research shows that the targeted provision of information has an independent impact on opinion change within a group, which can be considered separately from mere social conformity [s16]. An ally not only provides social backing but can also introduce new arguments, facts, or observations into the discussion that the majority may have overlooked or that were ignored in the process of groupthink. This new information can undermine the basis of the majority opinion and prompt other previously silent group members to reflect. One's own position is thus perceived not only as socially acceptable but also as substantively grounded.

The active search for support is a concrete action strategy. An effective way to mobilize such support is to discreetly approach individuals before a critical group situation. For instance, in a work team where a controversial new software is to be introduced, you might speak to a colleague whose technical judgment you value before the official meeting. An open, exploratory question like "I have some concerns about the compatibility of the new system with our existing processes. What do you think based on your experience?" is far more effective than the demanding question "Are you against it too?". Such an approach creates a space for honest exchange without immediately placing the person on one side. Often, it turns out that others share similar doubts but have also been hesitant to voice them. This phenomenon is a direct antidote to pluralistic ignorance, where many secretly agree but remain silent out of fear of isolation.

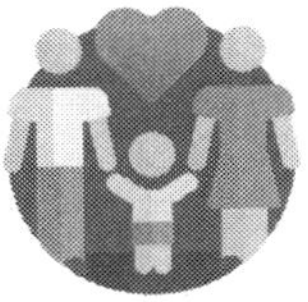

An ally does not need to fully share your position. Even a person who supports only partial aspects of your criticism can steer the discussion in a more constructive direction. If someone in the meeting about the software says, "I am generally in favor of the new software, but the point about compatibility is valid and should be thoroughly examined before a final decision," this already represents a significant strengthening of your position. This partial support signals to the group that your concerns are not unfounded and compels the proponents to engage with them argumentatively rather than dismissing the objection outright. The focus shifts from the person of the critic to the substantive issue. This dynamic allows you to present your arguments without having to constantly defend against accusations of mere obstructionism. The presence of an ally thus transforms a potentially hostile confrontation into a collaborative problem-solving process that not only strengthens your own position but also enhances the quality of the final group decision.

Good to know

groupthink

A mode of thinking that occurs in groups with strong cohesion, where the pursuit of unanimity overshadows realistic appraisal of alternative courses of action. Critical questioning is often suppressed.

informational influence

The influence of a person through the arguments and information presented by others. Opinion change occurs from the conviction that the perspective of others is factually correct.

pluralistic ignorance

A situation in which the majority of group members privately reject a norm or opinion but mistakenly assume that most others accept it. This leads to no one daring to express their own dissenting opinion.

social conformity

The adjustment of one's behavior or opinion to the actual or assumed norms of a group. This adjustment often occurs to belong or because one views the group as a source of correct information.

social dynamic

Refers to the interacting forces and processes that determine the behavior and relationships among members of a group. It encompasses aspects such as leadership, communication, and the formation of opinions.

The Ally Effect: How an Ally Helps Resist Group Pressure

Conceptual breakdown of the psychological components that an ally contributes to strengthen individual resolve against group pressure.

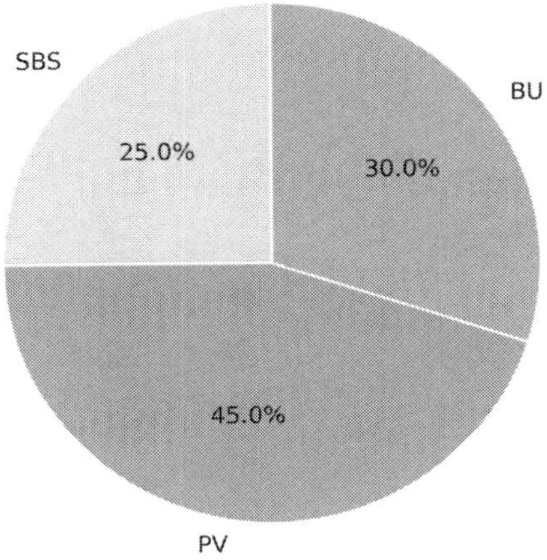

- BU: Breaking Unanimity
- PV: Psychological Validation
- SBS: Social Burden Sharing

This chart illustrates the key psychological mechanisms through which a single ally empowers an individual to resist conforming to a group. The largest factor, 'Psychological Validation' (45%), represents the immense relief and confidence gained from having one's own perception of reality confirmed, countering self-doubt. 'Breaking Unanimity' (30%) is the second crucial component; the mere presence of a dissenting voice shatters the illusion of a monolithic and infallible majority, making it psychologically easier to voice a different opinion. Finally, 'Social Burden Sharing' (25%) reflects the reduced fear of isolation and social reprisal. The perceived social cost of non-conformity is no longer on one individual but is shared, making the act of resistance far less intimidating. Please note that these percentages are conceptual estimates intended to illustrate the fundamental principles of social support. The actual impact of each factor can vary depending on the specific situation, the individuals involved, and the nature of the group.

2. 3 Questioning Obedience to Authorities

Obedience to authority is a foundation of social order. It ensures functioning processes in both professional and societal contexts, yet blind compliance carries significant dangers. The consequences range from personal moral conflicts to harmful group decisions and even overt abuse of power. This chapter reveals the criteria for distinguishing legitimate from illegitimate claims to authority. It analyzes the psychological barriers that hinder autonomous action and describes the path from internal conflict to justified dissent. Mastering this competence is the key to personal integrity and responsible action within any hierarchy.

The highest form of dissent is not mere refusal to obey, but the conscious assumption of responsibility for a better outcome.

“*He who does not punish evil commands that it be done.*”

Leonardo da Vinci

The Notebooks of Leonardo da Vinci (1883)

Translated as 'He who does not punish evil commands it to be done,' this quote powerfully addresses the moral responsibility of individuals in the face of authority. In the context of obedience studies, such as Milgram's experiments, it highlights the dilemma of the participant. By obeying an authority figure who commands a harmful act, the individual becomes complicit. The failure to defy an unjust command is, in itself, an act that permits evil to occur, forcing a deep reflection on personal responsibility versus deference to authority.

2.3.1 Recognizing Illegitimate Authority Claims

The distinction between legitimate and illegitimate authority claims is based on the source and scope of the respective authority. Legitimate authority relies on verifiable foundations such as expertise, a legally defined role, or societal consensus. In contrast, illegitimate claims lack this foundation and often rely on presumption, manipulation, or the abuse of a position. Recognizing such claims requires a conscious analysis of the situation and the individuals involved.

A first indicator for evaluation is competence. A person claiming authority should possess demonstrable expertise or relevant experience in the respective field. If these qualifications are absent, the claim should be critically questioned. Genuine experts can logically justify their arguments and are generally open to factual inquiries. In contrast, individuals with insufficient competence often respond evasively, aggressively, or attempt to stifle discussions by referring to their supposed position. A critical examination of qualifications or seeking a second, independent opinion are effective means to clarify the situation.

Another characteristic is the context-dependence of authority. Legitimation is almost always tied to a specific context. A police officer has the authority to issue commands in traffic as part of their official duties, but not in the medical treatment of a patient in a hospital. Illegitimate claims often arise when a person attempts to transfer their authority from one area to another, unrelated area. A supervisor who uses their professional position to demand personal favors from employees that go far beyond the employment contract exceeds the limits of their legitimate jurisdiction. The instruction itself may seem harmless, but the claim to be able to issue it is illegitimate, as it is based on an abuse of the professional hierarchy for personal purposes.

The nature of the instruction itself also provides crucial clues. Instructions that contradict ethical or legal norms are never legitimized by authority. No position justifies the request for illegal actions, harm to others, or the violation of fundamental moral principles. Special caution is warranted when the instructions are associated with manipulative tactics. These include, among others, the imposition of excessive time pressure, the social isolation of the affected person to prevent interaction with others, or appeals to loyalty and obedience that aim to suppress critical reflection. The demand for absolute confidentiality can also be a warning signal, as it seeks to remove the action from social control and evaluation.

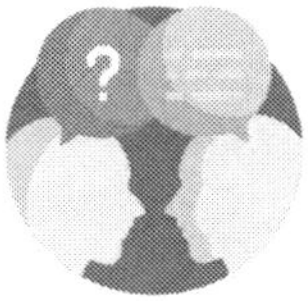

A close look at the motives of the authority figure can also be revealing. Does the instruction serve a comprehensible, factual goal that aligns with the role of the authority figure? Or does it primarily serve personal advantage, power demonstration, or the satisfaction of personal needs at the expense of others? Legitimate authority operates within defined goals and duties, while illegitimate claims are often driven by selfish or irrational motives.

In summary, illegitimate authority claims can be recognized through a systematic examination of several factors. The following points can serve as analytical tools:
- **Lack of competence:** The claim is disproportionate to the demonstrable knowledge and abilities of the person.
- **Context overreach:** Authority is exercised outside its legitimate scope.
- **Illegitimate or immoral content:** The instruction calls for actions that violate laws, ethical principles, or the rights of others.
- **Manipulative communication:** Pressure, emotional blackmail, or isolation are used to enforce obedience.
- **Self-serving motives:** The instruction does not serve a factual or communal purpose but primarily the personal advantage of the authority figure.

The ability to interpret these signals is a form of maturity. It not only protects one's integrity but also helps to prevent abuse of power in social and professional contexts. It is a conscious cognitive process that counters the automated impulse to obey with a rational assessment.

Good to know

Abuse of Power

The exploitation of a formal or informal power position to pursue personal goals that contradict the duties and responsibilities associated with that position.

Cognitive Process

The conscious thought process in which an instruction from an authority is not automatically followed but analyzed regarding its legitimacy, meaning, and consequences.

Context Overreach

A warning signal for illegitimate exercise of power, where an authority figure applies their valid authority in one area to a situation or topic for which they have no jurisdiction.

Legitimation

The social or psychological recognition that grants a person or institution the right to issue instructions and expect obedience. Without this recognition from subordinates, a claim to power remains purely formal.

Social Control

A mechanism through which the behavior of authority figures is regulated and aligned with recognized norms by public opinion or evaluation by other group members.

Indicators of Illegitimate Authority

Estimated frequency of key warning signs in situations of questionable authority.

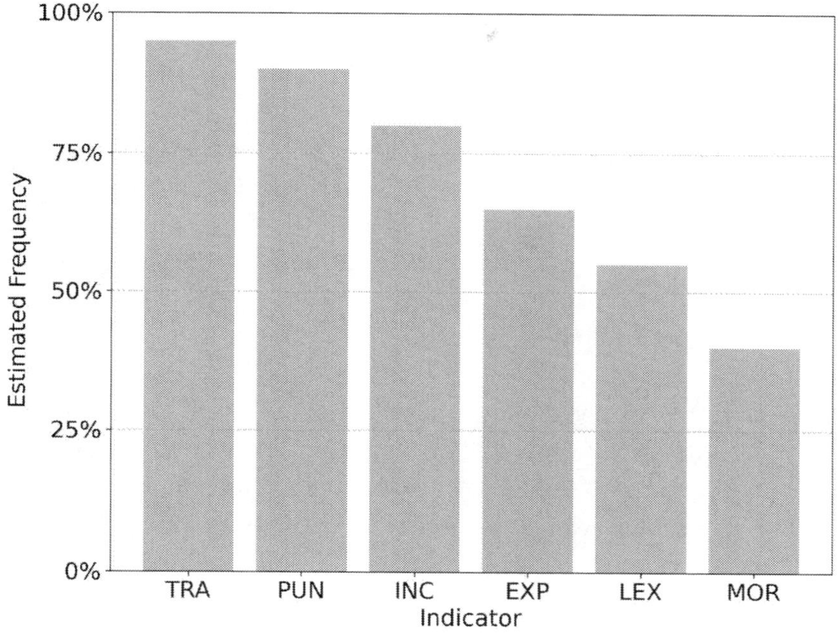

EXP: Exploitation for Gain
LEX: Lack of Expertise
PUN: Punishment of Dissent
INC: Inconsistent Rules
MOR: Moral/Ethical Violations
TRA: Lack of Transparency

The chart illustrates a conceptual model of common indicators that may signal an illegitimate claim to authority. High-frequency indicators such as 'Lack of Transparency' and 'Punishment of Dissent' are often the most immediate and pervasive signs. They create an environment of uncertainty and fear, which is fundamental to maintaining control without legitimate grounds. Mid-range indicators like 'Inconsistent Rules' and 'Exploitation' further erode trust and fairness. While 'Moral/Ethical Violations' are shown as less frequent, their presence is a severe and often undeniable sign of illegitimacy. It is important to note that these values are conceptual estimates designed to illustrate these principles, as the actual frequency can vary greatly depending on the specific context and group.

2.3.2 Strategies for Strengthening Personal Responsibility

The ability to identify illegitimate claims of authority is a prerequisite for independent action. The subsequent step is to solidify personal responsibility so that it withstands the pressure to obey. Under the influence of an authority, individuals tend to view themselves merely as executing tools and transfer the responsibility for the consequences of their actions to the commanding person. This psychological mechanism, known as "agentic shift," temporarily relieves the individual but can lead to morally questionable or harmful actions. Strengthening personal responsibility aims to consciously break through this mental state and regain one's role as an actively acting and deciding person.

An effective mental tool for this is the anticipation of future emotions. Instead of merely reacting to the immediate pressure of the situation, one shifts the focus to the long-term consequences for one's self-image. Studies suggest that a sense of responsibility and potential regret felt during the execution of a task increases the likelihood of disobedience to a harmful directive [s17]. This insight can be proactively utilized. Before taking an action that causes discomfort, ask yourself: "How will I feel about this decision in a month or a year? Will I be proud of my integrity or regret my capitulation?" This mental time travel helps to weigh the short-term desire for conformity or the fear of sanctions against the long-term preservation of one's moral values. The focus shifts from external authority to the inner moral compass.

Authorities often use goals or incentives to promote compliance with directives [s17]. A conscious strategy is to mentally separate these elements and consider the core of the directive in isolation. A department head asks their team to slightly "optimize" sales figures for the quarterly report to secure an important bonus for everyone. The justification ("We are securing jobs and rewarding our hard work") and the incentive (the bonus payment) obscure the core of the directive: the falsification of data. By decoupling the actual action from its supposed justification and the promised reward, the moral substance of the request becomes clearer. The critical evaluation of the actual act can then occur free from manipulative framing.

The feeling of having no other choice is a common accompaniment to blind obedience. However, experiments show that the mere possibility of a free choice increases the willingness to disobey [s17]. The realization that there is almost always a choice – even if the alternatives are unpleasant – is a crucial step toward taking responsibility. The decision to follow a directive to avoid negative consequences such as termination or social exclusion is also a choice. This cognitive reframing, shifting from "I had to do it" to "I chose to do it under the given circumstances," restores control over the situation. It makes one's involvement visible and forces engagement with the motives behind one's decision.

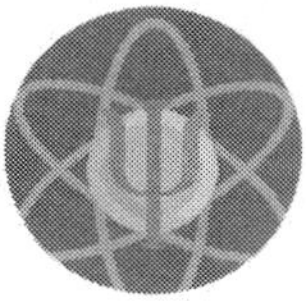

Personal disposition also influences the willingness to take responsibility. Individuals with a naturally lower acceptance of authority are more likely to engage in prosocial disobedience, meaning they refuse directives that would harm others [s17]. However, this attitude can be trained. Purposeful yet moderate questioning of smaller, unproblematic directives in everyday life can serve as practice. Those who learn to express a reasoned dissent in low-risk situations build self-confidence and mental routines. This makes it easier to remain steadfast even in critical moments of high pressure. It is not about rejecting all authority but cultivating the ability to examine directives rationally rather than obeying automatically. Taking responsibility is thus not a passive state but an active cognitive process. It requires the mental anticipation of one's emotional reaction, the critical analysis of justifications, the conscious acknowledgment of one's freedom of choice, and the gradual practice of responsible behavior.

Good to know

Agentic Shift

A mental state described by Stanley Milgram in which a person no longer perceives themselves as an independently acting subject but as an instrument for executing the wishes of an authority figure. In this state, the moral evaluation of one's actions is suspended, and the focus is placed on the correct fulfillment of the directive.

Conformity

The adjustment of one's behavior or opinion to the perceived norms or behavior of a group. Unlike obedience, this adjustment often occurs without a direct command but arises from the desire to belong or not to stand out negatively.

Prosocial Disobedience

The conscious refusal to follow a directive from an authority that is deemed unethical or harmful to others. The motivation for this disobedience is not personal gain but the protection or well-being of third parties. Such behavior is often referred to as whistleblowing when it occurs in organizational contexts.

Effectiveness of Strategies to Take Responsibility

Perceived effectiveness of strategies to resist undue authority.

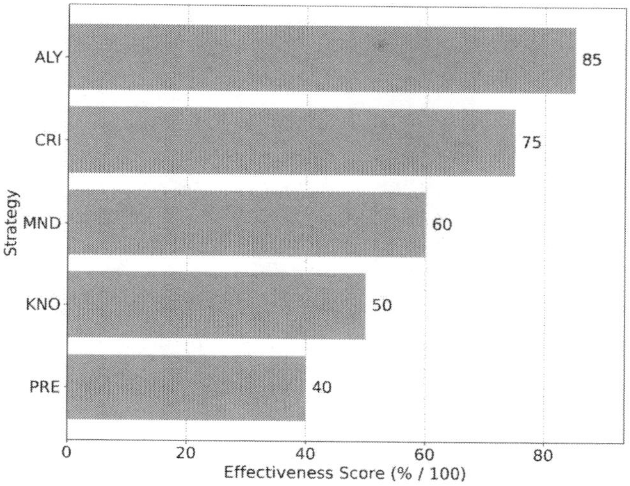

ALY: Seeking an Ally
CRI: Critical Thinking
KNO: Psychological Knowledge
MND: Mindfulness and Self-Awareness
PRE: Pre-Commitment to Values

The chart illustrates a comparison of different strategies aimed at strengthening personal responsibility, particularly in situations involving pressure from authority figures. The most effective strategy appears to be 'Seeking an Ally'. This aligns with classic social psychology findings, which show that the presence of even a single dissenting voice can dramatically reduce conformity and obedience. It breaks the illusion of universal consent and provides the social support needed to act on one's own convictions. 'Critical Thinking' and 'Mindfulness and Self-Awareness' also rank highly as powerful internal tools. They enable an individual to pause, evaluate the moral and logical implications of a command, and connect with their own values before acting. The data suggests that while internal preparedness is crucial, external social support can be the most decisive factor in the moment of pressure. Please note that these values are principled estimates designed to represent the relative effectiveness of these psychological strategies based on established research in social psychology.

2.3.3 Practices of Constructive Dissent in Hierarchies

After personal responsibility has been strengthened and the decision to reject an instruction has been made, the implementation takes the form of constructive dissent. Such dissent is not open rebellion but a targeted communication effort aimed at correcting a problematic decision while maintaining the working relationship with the authority figure. Its effectiveness largely depends on preparation, word choice, and the chosen context.

The foundation of any constructive dissent is solid, factual argumentation. Instead of acting out of an emotional reaction, this practice requires a conscious distancing from one's own outrage or fear. The criticism is directed not against the authority figure as an individual but solely against the content or potential consequences of an instruction. A dissent expressed based on verifiable facts, data, or logical conclusions shifts the discussion from a personal confrontation to an objective level. This undermines the accusation of mere insubordination and frames the dissenter as an engaged and thoughtful actor. Preparation involves gathering all relevant information that supports one's concerns and mentally anticipating possible counterarguments.

The nature of communication is crucial for success. Accusatory phrases like "Your plan is flawed" or "You cannot order this" provoke a defensive stance and lead the authority figure to retreat to their formal power position. More effective is the use of "I-messages", which frame concerns as personal perceptions. A statement like "I have concerns about the legal permissibility of this approach" or "I see a potential safety risk for the team if we skip this step" is less confrontational. It opens a space for dialogue rather than hardening positions. The situation is comparable to a project manager receiving the instruction to use a cheaper but inadequately tested component. Instead of outright rejecting the instruction, they could articulate their concerns specifically: "I have reviewed the specifications of the new component and see a measurable risk to product lifespan under continuous load due to the lower material density. May I present an alternative calculation that also considers long-term warranty costs?" This approach directly links dissent to a proposed solution and demonstrates loyalty to the overarching goals of the company, not to a single potentially flawed instruction.

The timing and location of dissent are also strategic components. A dissent expressed in front of a whole group or in a public meeting can be perceived by the authority figure as a public attack on their competence and position. This increases the pressure to save face and enforce the instruction at all costs. A one-on-one conversation is often the better choice. It creates a confidential atmosphere where concerns can be openly discussed without fear of social devaluation. Additionally, seeking allies can strengthen one's position. Solomon Asch's experiments showed that even a single ally can significantly reduce conformity_pressure. In a work context, this means discreetly talking to trusted colleagues beforehand to determine if concerns are shared. An objection raised collectively or on behalf of several individuals carries more weight and distributes the perceived risk across multiple shoulders.

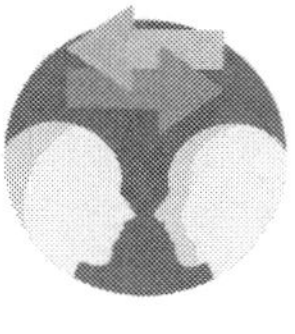

Constructive dissent does not end with the expression of concerns. It should always be accompanied by the offer to actively contribute to a better solution. Those who point out problems should ideally be able to present well-thought-out alternatives. This signals that the aim is not to refuse work but to optimize the outcome. After a conversation, it is also advisable to summarize the key points and agreed next steps in a brief, neutral email. This serves documentation, prevents misunderstandings, and underscores the professionalism of the approach. In summary, the process can be divided into the following steps:

- Formulate concerns factually and data-driven to decouple criticism from the personal.
- Communicate dissent as an "I-message" to avoid a defensive reaction.
- Prefer a one-on-one conversation over a public forum to avoid embarrassing the authority.
- Propose concrete, well-thought-out alternatives to position oneself as solution-oriented.

Through these practices, potentially destructive disobedience transforms into a constructive contribution that can protect organizations from poor decisions and foster a culture of psychological safety, where concerns can be expressed without fear.

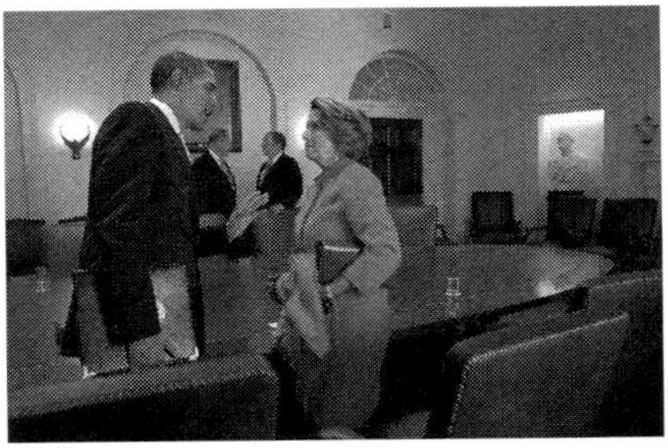

one-on-one meeting [i11]

Good to know

Authority Figure

A person who is attributed the ability to give instructions and expect obedience due to their formal position, knowledge, or personal charisma. The willingness to follow an authority figure strongly depends on the perceived legitimacy of their power.

Conformity Pressure

The often unspoken pressure exerted by a group to align one's opinion or behavior with the prevailing group norm. In the face of authority, this pressure can be intensified, as the group often tends to rally behind the authority figure.

Insubordination

Refers to the conscious refusal to follow a perceived legitimate instruction from a superior. From a social psychological perspective, the fear of being accused of insubordination can be a strong barrier that prevents individuals from questioning morally or factually questionable instructions.

Psychological Safety

A group or organizational climate in which members feel safe to take interpersonal risks, such as expressing concerns or admitting mistakes, without fearing negative consequences. It is a crucial prerequisite to prevent blind obedience.

Effectiveness of Dissent in Hierarchies

Shows how the likelihood of a positive outcome increases with the constructiveness of the dissent.

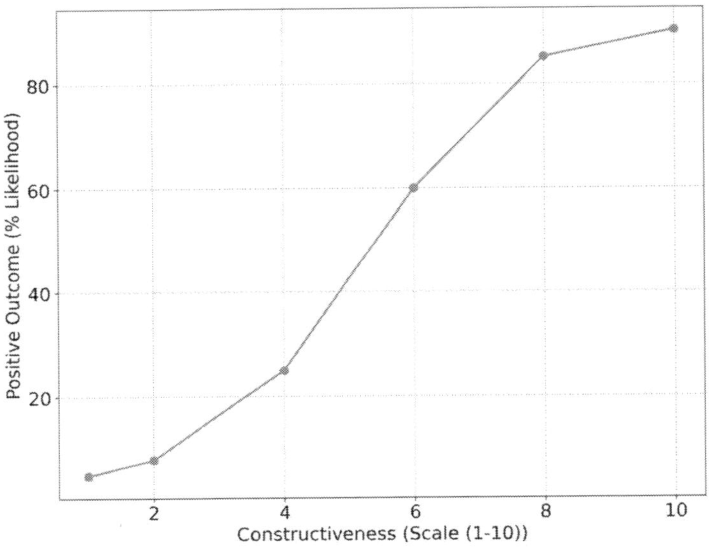

This chart illustrates the relationship between the method of expressing dissent and its probable success within a hierarchical structure. At the lower end of the x-axis, where dissent is destructive or passive-aggressive (e.g., personal attacks, sabotage), the likelihood of a positive outcome is minimal. Authorities tend to react defensively, shutting down communication and reinforcing their position. As the approach becomes more constructive—moving from simple questioning to proposing well-reasoned, solution-oriented alternatives—the probability of success rises dramatically. The curve flattens at the top, suggesting that highly constructive, collaborative dissent consistently yields the best results. The key takeaway is that how one voices disagreement is critical; a focus on shared goals and solutions, rather than mere opposition, is far more effective at influencing authority and achieving positive change. The data shown are estimates intended to illustrate this fundamental principle of organizational dynamics.

Concrete Advice

- Request to receive any ethically or legally questionable instructions in writing for the protection of all parties involved.
- Encourage the authority figure to engage in a mental role reversal by asking, 'How would you decide in my position, bound by my professional duties?'
- Frame your objection in the service of a higher principle by relating your concerns to the long-term reputation of the organization or shared values.
- Examine an instruction by imagining it came from someone you respect unconditionally—if your doubts persist, the issue lies within the instruction itself.
- Inquire specifically about what precedent your actions would set for future similar situations within the team or organization.
- Conduct a critical conversation deliberately in a room where corporate values or ethical guidelines are visibly displayed on the wall, to involve them as silent witnesses.
- Do not refuse the entire task, but only the one, untenable aspect, and offer to implement the rest with even greater commitment.
- Redefine obedience for yourself, not as following a person, but as loyalty to the rules and goals that this person should ideally represent.
- Ask about the origin of a questionable instruction to clarify whether the authority figure is acting under pressure and may be open to a collaborative approach.
- Utilize a 'question of jurisdiction' by politely clarifying, 'Does the responsibility for the potential negative consequences of this action also fall within your area of responsibility?'

Review - 2. Social Influence: Persuasion Strategies and Conformity Pressure

Understanding social influence begins with the realization that communication rarely occurs on a single level. Rather, we constantly operate within a tension between factual argumentation and emotional-heuristic influence. In practice, this means a continuous diagnosis of your counterpart and the situation: Is your conversation partner motivated and capable of engaging deeply with facts, or are they distracted, in a hurry, or emotionally biased? If you wish to facilitate a long-term, well-founded decision, such as the implementation of a new strategy within a team, the central route is indispensable. Prepare not only data and logical arguments but also consciously create the mental space for their processing: Schedule a meeting that allows sufficient time, send documents in advance, and actively invite critical questions. Conversely, if you face the challenge of capturing attention in a stimulus-saturated environment—such as a trade fair or a social media feed—peripheral cues are your key to success. A compelling image, a quote from a respected authority, or an emotionally appealing slogan can open the door to being perceived for a deeper message. The art lies in strategically combining these routes without becoming manipulative.

The most effective principles of influence, such as reciprocity, social proof, or likability, often exert their power below the threshold of consciousness. However, true mastery does not lie in mechanical application but in authentic integration into your actions. Instead of making a calculated "gift" before a request, offer selflessly help or valuable information in advance. This builds a genuine relationship, and the resulting impulse for reciprocation is an organic consequence, not a forced reaction. The same applies to social proof: Instead of merely advertising with anonymous user numbers, highlight success stories from customers who resemble your target audience in their challenges and goals. Identification creates a much stronger persuasive power than an abstract number. The greatest challenge with these techniques is maintaining one's integrity. Always ask yourself: Would my counterpart still comply with my request if they fully understood the psychological strategy being applied? If the answer is "Yes," you are acting persuasively. If it is "No," you are acting manipulatively.

The ability to exert influence requires, as a counterpart, the competence to withstand unwanted pressure and maintain one's judgment. This is particularly true in group and hierarchical situations. If you sense that a majority opinion or a directive from an authority figure causes you discomfort, the first step is to pause. Resist the impulse to remain silent out of fear of isolation or to react emotionally in protest. The most effective strategy is often to translate your gut feeling into a constructive, factual question. Do not express your doubts as an accusation ("That is wrong!"), but as a desire for clarification ("I want to ensure that I have understood all aspects. Could we discuss the potential risks of Option A again?"). This approach depersonalizes the criticism and forces the group to substantiate their position argumentatively, rather than labeling you as a troublemaker. Additionally, do not confront an authority figure publicly; instead, seek a one-on-one conversation. This preserves your counterpart's face and dramatically increases the likelihood of an open discussion. Actively and discreetly seeking an ally in advance can further facilitate this process and provide you with the necessary backing.

Ultimately, the strategies outlined here culminate in an overarching ability: the conscious design of social interactions. It is not about learning a repertoire of tricks but about recognizing and navigating the psychological currents in every communication. Whether you are presenting an idea, leading a team, negotiating a salary, or resisting an unethical directive—there is always a balance to be struck between logical persuasion, emotional connection, and the management of group dynamics. Applying these principles not only makes you a more persuasive communicator but, above all, a more autonomous and responsible actor in any social structure. Begin by observing these dynamics in your daily life—this first step of awareness is the most important on the path to mastery.

3. Group Psychology in Practice: Shaping Dynamics and Collaboration

Why do some teams fail despite excellent individual performances, while others exceed expectations and achieve extraordinary results? The answer lies not in the abilities of the members, but in the invisible forces that operate between them. Groups follow their own laws, which can be both beneficial and detrimental to shared goals. Understanding these mechanisms allows for the unlocking of potential, overcoming obstacles, and creating constructive working relationships. This chapter demonstrates how insights from group psychology can be effectively utilized to transform a collection of individuals into a functioning team.

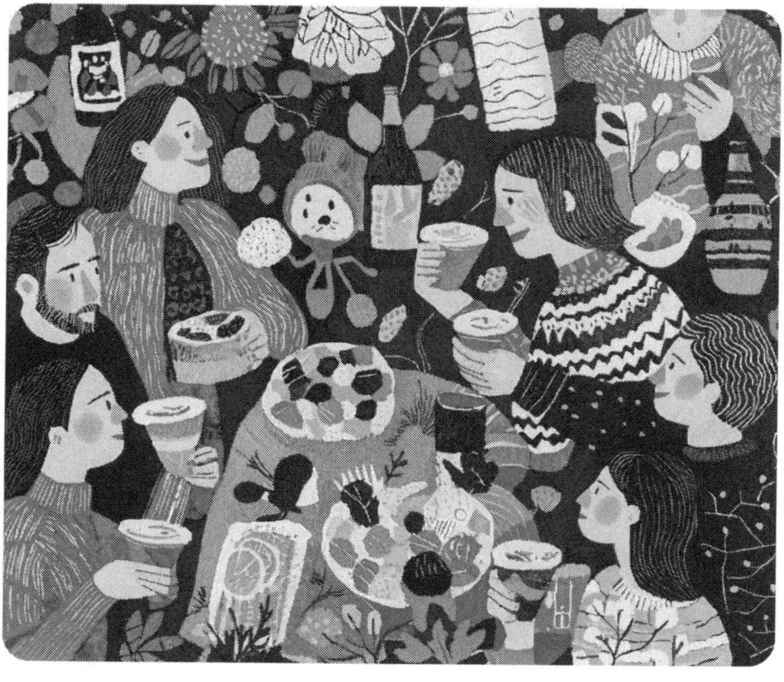

Group Dynamics: Fiascos & Triumphs

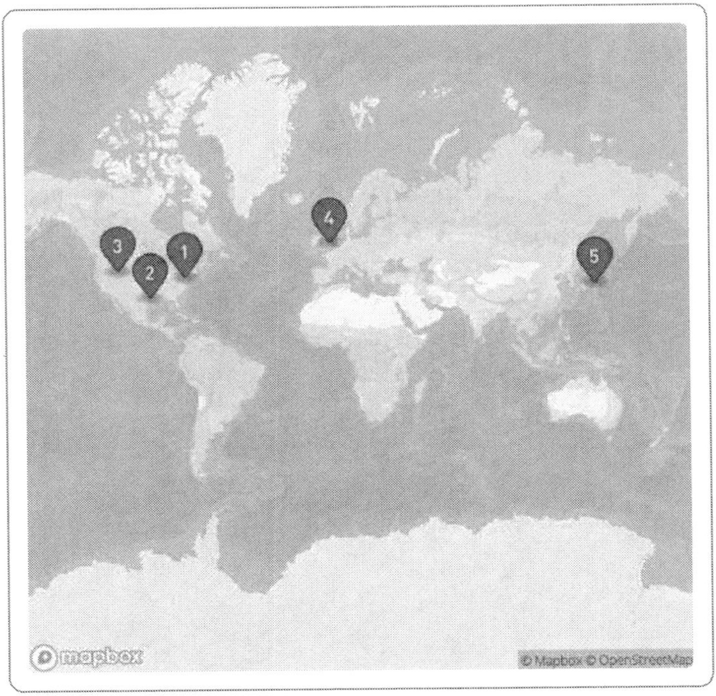

A map highlighting historical examples of groupthink failures and successful team collaborations.

1 **The White House: Bay of Pigs Invasion**

GROUPTHINK: In 1961, President John F. Kennedy's advisory group planned the failed Bay of Pigs invasion. The group dynamic suffered from an illusion of invulnerability, self-censorship of doubts, and direct pressure on dissenters. This desire for consensus led the group to overlook fatal flaws in the plan, resulting in a major political and military fiasco.

2 **NASA Mission Control: Apollo 13 Crisis**

SUCCESSFUL COLLABORATION: In 1970, an explosion crippled the Apollo 13 spacecraft. The Mission Control team in Houston demonstrated exceptional problem-solving. They abandoned hierarchy, fostered open communication, and leveraged diverse expertise under immense pressure. Their mantra, 'Failure is not an option,' drove a collaborative effort that safely returned the astronauts to Earth.

3 **Morton Thiokol HQ: Challenger Disaster**

GROUPTHINK: The 1986 Space Shuttle Challenger disaster is a tragic case of groupthink. Engineers at contractor Morton Thiokol warned that the O-rings could fail in cold weather. However, management under pressure from NASA to meet launch deadlines, overruled these technical concerns. The group dynamic prioritized the launch schedule over safety, leading to catastrophic failure.

4 **Bletchley Park: Enigma Codebreakers**

SUCCESSFUL COLLABORATION: During WWII, a diverse team of mathematicians, linguists, and engineers at Bletchley Park collaborated to break the German Enigma code. They fostered a culture of intellectual freedom and cross-disciplinary problem-solving, creating innovative techniques and machines. Their success significantly shortened the war and saved countless lives.

5 **Fukushima Daiichi Nuclear Power Plant**

GROUPTHINK: The 2011 Fukushima disaster was exacerbated by a culture of groupthink. A rigid hierarchical structure, deference to authority, and an unwillingness to question assumptions meant that warnings about the plant's vulnerability to tsunamis were ignored for years. During the crisis, this led to slow and ineffective decision-making, compounding the disaster's severity.

3. 1 Increasing Group Performance and Productivity

Collaboration in groups holds significant potential but also specific risks. Often, collective performance falls short of the capabilities of individual members. Valuable synergies remain untapped, while inefficient processes and communication problems hinder productivity and lead to frustration. This chapter illuminates the psychological mechanisms behind performance losses and unused potential. It addresses how the targeted design of tasks, interactions, and communication structures can strengthen individual accountability and enable the emergence of collective intelligence. The following sections provide the psychological tools to systematically optimize group work and achieve measurable success.

> *True group performance arises not merely from the sum of individual contributions, but through the conscious design of structures that make personal responsibility visible while also enabling safe, synergistic interaction.*

> *Assist a man in raising a burden - but do not assist him in laying it down.*

Pythagoras

The Symbols
Symbol 11

This ancient saying provides a profound metaphor for effective teamwork and the enhancement of group performance. True assistance empowers the group and its members to achieve their goals ('raising a burden'). However, fostering dependency or doing the work for others ('assisting in laying it down') ultimately weakens the group's capabilities and long-term productivity. The goal of collaboration should be to build collective strength, not to encourage social loafing.

3.1.1 Methods to Prevent Social Loafing

To counteract the phenomenon of social loafing, several application-oriented strategies exist that directly address the psychological causes of this effect. The core of these methods lies in changing the conditions under which group work takes place to enhance individual motivation and accountability.

A primary approach is to increase the Identifiability and measurability of individual performance. Social loafing occurs primarily when the personal contribution is lost in the overall result of the group and is no longer attributable. To prevent this, tasks should be structured so that the contributions of each member remain visible. This can be achieved, among other things, by breaking down a large group goal into clearly defined, distinct sub-tasks assigned to individual persons or small teams. For instance, in the creation of a research report, one member could be responsible for literature research, another for data collection, and a third for statistical analysis. Although the individual results will later be combined into a whole, they remain recognizable and evaluable as personal achievements. Evaluating individual performance, in addition to assessing the overall result, reinforces this effect. Regular, brief progress reports in which each member presents their completed tasks and next steps also create transparency and a form of social control that fosters engagement.

The perceived importance and personal meaning of the task also influence performance willingness. People are less likely to loaf when they view their task as significant and their contribution as essential to the group's success. Leaders or project managers can support this by clearly communicating the purpose and relevance of the project and demonstrating how each individual's specific contribution contributes to the success of the whole. Motivation increases when the task is challenging yet achievable and aligns with the employee's abilities. A task that poses a certain challenge mobilizes more cognitive and motivational resources than an underwhelming routine task. Furthermore, granting autonomy in executing assigned tasks enhances the sense of personal responsibility and ownership.

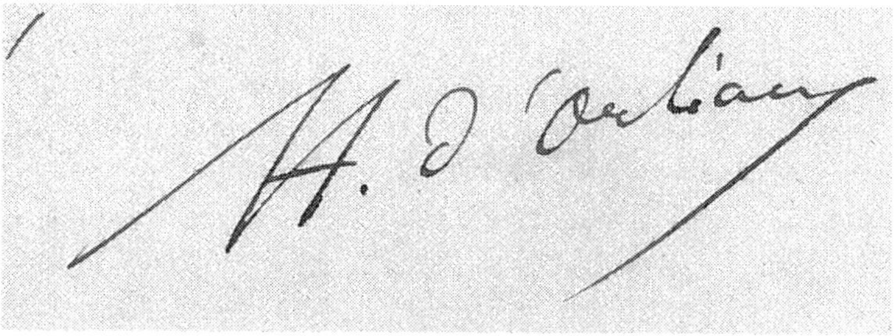

Identifiability [i12]

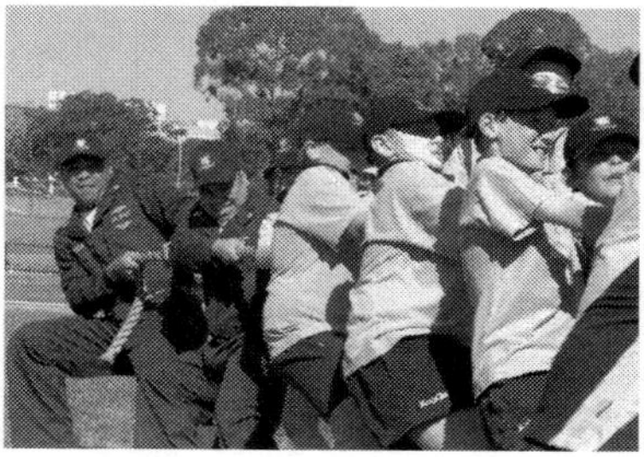

group cohesion [i13]

Another factor is group cohesion, which refers to the solidarity and "we-feeling" within the group. In groups with strong social bonds and mutual respect, members do not want to disappoint one another. The desire to make a positive impression on colleagues they value counteracts social loafing. Team-building measures, the establishment of shared norms and values, and the emphasis on common goals rather than internal competition can strengthen cohesion. When group members see themselves as part of a high-performing and mutually supportive team, the likelihood that individuals will reduce their efforts decreases.

The size of the group itself is a simple yet effective lever. As the number of members increases, the potential for social loafing rises, as anonymity grows and the individual contribution becomes proportionally smaller. The likelihood that someone thinks, "My effort doesn't matter here anyway," increases. Therefore, workgroups should be kept as small as possible without losing the necessary diversity of skills and perspectives for task completion. For complex projects requiring a large number of people, structuring into smaller, autonomous subgroups with clear interfaces and responsibilities is advisable.

In summary, the most effective methods can be consolidated into a few points aimed at reducing anonymity and creating personal relevance:

- Clear assignment of individual tasks with defined responsibilities.
- Visibility of individual contributions, for example, through separate reports or personal presentations of work results.

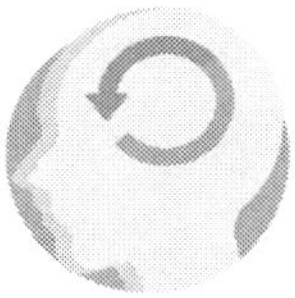

- Emphasis on the personal relevance and indispensability of each contribution to achieving the group goal.
- Promotion of a high degree of group cohesion through shared goals and mutual appreciation.
- Establishment of clear and objective performance standards against which the group and each member can measure themselves.
- Optimization of group size; smaller groups are generally less susceptible to social loafing.

The consistent application of these principles alters the dynamics of collaboration. It shifts the focus from an anonymous collective to a community of identifiable individuals who feel responsible for their specific contributions and recognize their necessity for collective success.

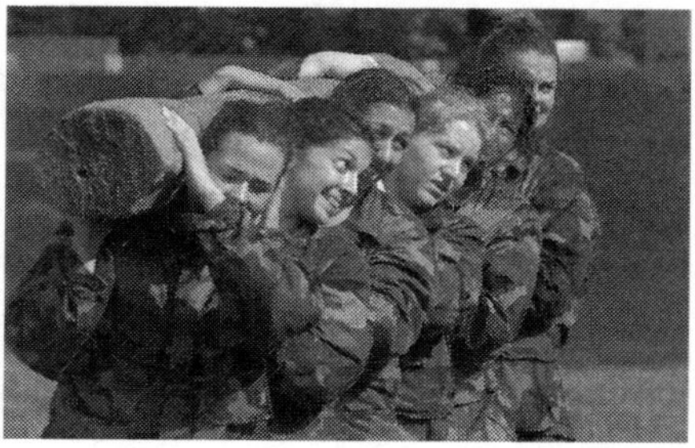

Team building [i14]

Good to know

Anonymity

The state in which a person does not feel perceived as a single, identifiable individual within a group. This felt invisibility can lead to deindividuation, where personal responsibility decreases.

Identifiability

The principle that a member's performance is visible to the group and personally attributable to them. This activates a state of heightened self-awareness, leading individuals to align their behavior more closely with personal or social norms.

Social Control

Refers to the informal and formal mechanisms through which a group regulates the behavior of its members and ensures adherence to norms. It operates through mutual observation and the subtle pressure to meet the expectations of other members.

Social Loafing

Refers to the tendency of individuals to exert less effort on collective tasks because they assume others will do the work or because they want to avoid bearing the main burden alone. This effect is often unconscious and strongly depends on the perceived fairness within the group.

Effectiveness of Methods Against Social Loafing

Estimated increase in group productivity by method

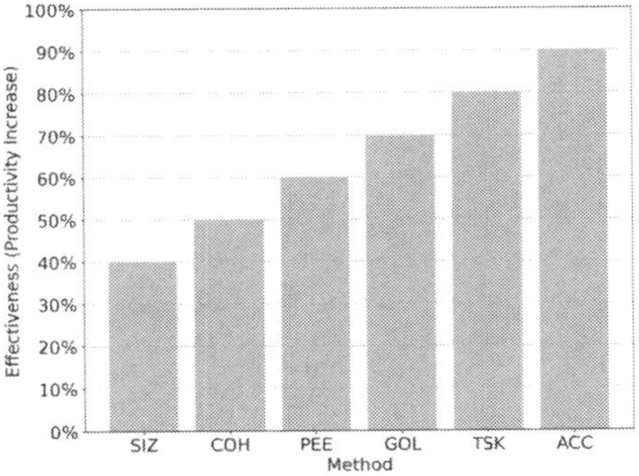

ACC: Individual Accountability

GOL: Specific Group Goals

SIZ: Smaller Group Size

COH: Group Cohesion

PEE: Peer Evaluation

TSK: Task Meaningfulness

This chart illustrates the estimated effectiveness of various methods in combating social loafing and increasing group productivity. It's important to note that these figures are principled estimates designed to demonstrate the relative impact of each strategy, not data from a single, specific study. The most effective methods are those that directly address the root causes of social loafing: anonymity and a lack of personal investment. 'Individual Accountability' is highly effective because it makes each person's contribution visible, eliminating the ability to hide in the group. Similarly, increasing 'Task Meaningfulness' gives members a personal reason to invest effort, making the work intrinsically rewarding. Methods like setting 'Specific Group Goals' and implementing 'Peer Evaluation' provide structure and social incentives, proving moderately to highly effective. They clarify expectations and introduce a layer of mutual responsibility. Structural and social-environmental factors such as 'Group Cohesion' and using a 'Smaller Group Size' are also beneficial. Smaller groups naturally increase visibility and responsibility, while cohesive groups can foster a sense of team identity and mutual obligation, though this is slightly less impactful on its own than direct accountability measures. The conclusion is that a multi-faceted approach, combining accountability with motivational and structural changes, is most likely to maximize group performance.

3.1.2 Promotion of synergy effects and group intelligence

The promotion of synergy effects and collective intelligence aims to achieve an outcome that exceeds the sum of potential individual performances. While the avoidance of social loafing ensures that individual contributions are not lost, the focus here is on creating an environment where these contributions reinforce each other and merge into new, higher-quality solutions. This process does not occur by chance; it requires the conscious design of interaction and thinking processes within the group. The foundation for this is the realization that the cognitive capacity of a team depends less on the average or maximum intelligence of its members and more on the quality of social interactions.

A starting point for unleashing group intelligence is the establishment of psychological safety. Members must have the confidence to express unconventional ideas, concerns, and even mistakes openly, without fearing negative personal consequences such as ridicule or a devaluation of their competence. If this safety is not present, individuals tend to self-censor. They withhold potentially valuable but risky or divergent thoughts to avoid conformity pressure. This limits the pool of available ideas to the lowest common denominator. A leader can actively cultivate psychological safety by making their own uncertainties or mistakes transparent and deliberately seeking counterarguments to their own proposals. This signals that critical questioning and intellectual engagement are welcome and valued as strengths rather than attacks. This state reduces the cognitive load created by social anxiety and frees mental resources for creative and analytical tasks.

On this basis, the cognitive diversity of a group can be effectively utilized. Synergy arises precisely from the productive friction of different perspectives, knowledge levels, and problem-solving approaches. A homogeneous group that quickly reaches a consensus risks overlooking relevant aspects and falling into the trap of groupthink. To counteract this, targeted techniques to promote constructive dissent can be implemented. One method involves institutionalizing and rotating the role of the "Advocatus Diaboli" (Devil's Advocate). The assigned member has the explicit task of identifying the weaknesses of proposals, questioning assumptions, and developing alternative scenarios. Since this criticism is a designated role and not a personal opinion, it becomes depersonalized, reducing the likelihood of defensive reactions. This forces the group to sharpen its own arguments and make its solutions more robust.

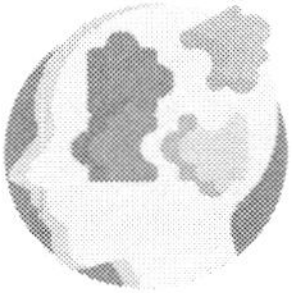

However, the mere existence of good ideas and constructive criticism does not automatically lead to better group outcomes. Clearly defined processes are needed to structure, consolidate, and translate this potential into a tangible decision or solution. This is where targeted team development interventions come into play, understood as systematic measures to improve team processes. Such interventions are most effective when tailored to the specific needs and developmental stage of the team and require the active participation of all members. Instead of general workshops, this may mean optimizing specific workflows. A team struggling to translate discussions into concrete actions might introduce a structured decision-making process. This could involve a phase of silent, individual idea generation for each complex problem, followed by a moderated discussion round where all ideas are collected without immediate evaluation. Only in a third step are the collected proposals jointly analyzed, evaluated, and combined into an integrated solution. Such a process ensures that even more introverted members can contribute, and dominant voices do not prematurely steer the discussion in one direction. By documenting not only the final decision but also the examined alternatives and the reasons for their rejection, the team creates a knowledge base that improves future decisions and fosters collective learning.

In summary, group intelligence is a cultivated ability. It arises from a foundation of psychological safety, is fueled by the conscious use of cognitive diversity and constructive dissent, and is channeled through structured processes. The implementation of such frameworks and techniques, ideally as needs-based and participatory interventions, transforms a collection of individual fighters into a synergetic system capable of solving complex problems in ways that would be unattainable for a single member.

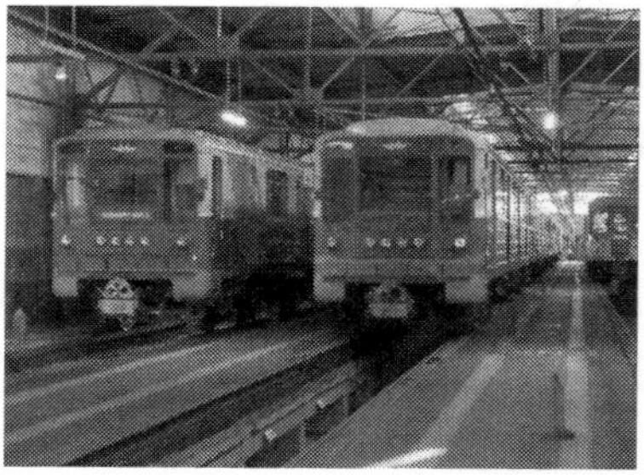

synergy effects [i15]

Good to know

Cognitive Diversity

Refers to the presence of different perspectives, knowledge backgrounds, and thinking styles within a group. This diversity is an important resource as it increases the likelihood of viewing a problem from multiple angles and finding a more comprehensive solution.

Collective Intelligence

Describes the ability of a group to act intelligently as a whole. It is a property that does not directly depend on the intelligence of individual members. Important factors for its emergence include a high social sensitivity of the members and an even distribution of speaking time.

Psychological Safety

Refers to the shared belief among team members that it is safe to take interpersonal risks. This means being able to express ideas, questions, or concerns without fear of punishment or humiliation. It is the foundation for learning behavior in teams.

Team Development Intervention

A planned measure aimed at improving the effectiveness of a team. Such measures focus on optimizing workflows, communication patterns, or role clarifications to enhance collaboration and achieve common goals.

Composition of Group Intelligence

Estimated contribution of different factors to a group's collective intelligence.

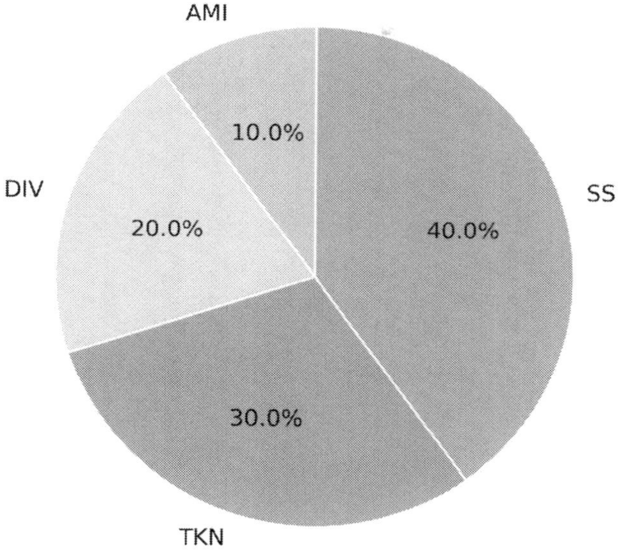

AMI: Average Member Intelligence
DIV: Cognitive Diversity
SS: Social Sensitivity
TKN: Equal Turn-Taking

This chart illustrates the estimated relative importance of various factors in determining a group's collective intelligence. It highlights that social dynamics are often more crucial than the sheer individual intelligence of the members. The largest component, 'Social Sensitivity' underscores the importance of empathy and the ability to interpret social cues. 'Equal Turn-Taking' demonstrates that balanced communication, preventing dominance by a few individuals, is vital for effective collaboration. 'Cognitive Diversity' contributes significantly by bringing varied perspectives and problem-solving approaches, which prevents groupthink and fosters innovation. Notably, 'Average Member Intelligence' has the smallest estimated impact, suggesting that a group of moderately intelligent but socially adept individuals can easily outperform a group of brilliant but poorly communicating experts. These values are conceptual estimates intended to illustrate the fundamental principles of group psychology and synergy.

3.1.3 Optimization of Communication Structures in the Team

Communication structures within a team establish the pathways through which information flows. These networks are not random; they significantly determine the speed and accuracy of information exchange, the effectiveness of problem-solving, and the satisfaction of members. Optimizing these structures requires an analysis of the prevailing tasks and goals, as different requirements favor various communication patterns. A fundamental distinction is made between centralized and decentralized networks. In centralized structures, such as the wheel or star pattern, all communication flows through a central person or position. This individual collects, filters, and distributes information to other members, who interact little or not at all directly with one another. In contrast, decentralized structures, such as the circular or fully connected model (total connectivity), allow for free communication among all or several members without a central intermediary.

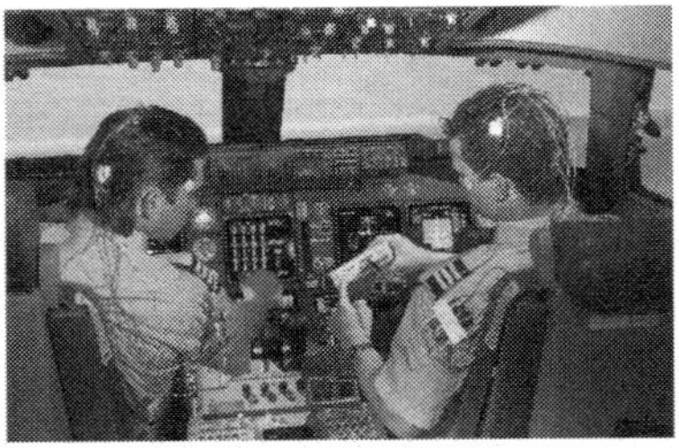

cognitive load [i16]

The choice of the appropriate network directly depends on the nature of the task. Centralized structures prove superior for simple, repetitive, or clearly defined tasks. The consolidation of communication in one person enables quick coordination and clear decision-making pathways, as the information flow remains manageable and is controlled from a single point. This minimizes redundancies and accelerates execution. However, this model has drawbacks: the central person can quickly become a bottleneck and is subject to high cognitive load. Peripheral members often feel less involved in the overall process, and their motivation and general satisfaction may decline, as they experience little autonomy and their contributions are filtered. Over time, this structure can be detrimental to the morale and innovation potential of the team.

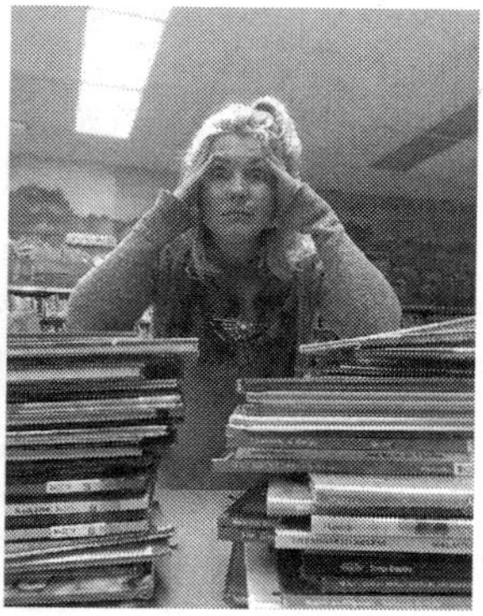

information overload [i17]

Decentralized networks unleash their strength in complex, ambiguous, and creative tasks that require diverse expertise and the integration of different perspectives. The free exchange of information among all members fosters the emergence of new ideas and allows for a more comprehensive problem analysis, improving the quality of results and decisions. The collective intelligence of the group, as described in the previous section, can flourish better in such an environment. The direct involvement of all members also promotes satisfaction, engagement, and a sense of shared responsibility. The downside is potentially lower efficiency in simple tasks. Without clear protocols, coordination can become chaotic, decision-making processes may slow down, and there is a risk of information overload, where distinguishing relevant from irrelevant messages becomes challenging.

Practical optimization, therefore, does not lie in rigid adherence to a single model but in the conscious and flexible design of communication pathways according to requirements. For instance, a team designing a new software architecture may benefit from a decentralized network in the initial phase, where all developers freely exchange ideas and concerns. Once the plan is established and it moves into the implementation phase, a more centralized structure with a lead developer as coordinator for the assignment and monitoring of programming tasks can enhance efficiency. The conscious adaptation of the structure to the respective project phase is a hallmark of high-performing teams.

To translate these theoretical models into practice, establishing clear communication protocols is helpful. These define which channels are used for which type of information and what expectations are attached to interactions. Such a protocol could regulate the following points:

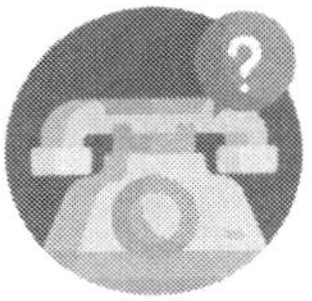

- **Channel Selection:** For urgent, action-required information, a direct messaging service is used; for general project updates, a shared channel in a collaboration tool; for in-depth discussions and decisions, a meeting is scheduled; formal documentation and reports are sent via email.
- **Meeting Structure:** Each meeting has a pre-communicated agenda, a set timeframe, and a moderator who guides the discussion. At the end, concrete action steps and responsibilities are recorded in the minutes to ensure accountability.
- **Information Flow in Decisions:** It is defined who must be consulted or merely informed for each type of decision. This prevents both the overlooking of relevant stakeholders and the unnecessary involvement of uninvolved persons.

By explicitly designing these structures and rules, the flow of information is channeled and adapted to the needs of the task. The team thus avoids friction losses, misunderstandings, and inefficient processes. Members gain clarity about their roles in the communication network, which improves collaboration and enhances collective performance.

Good to know

Cognitive Load

Describes the amount of mental effort a group member must expend to process information and manage tasks. Excessive load, such as from unstructured communication, can lead to errors, slower decisions, and a decline in overall team performance.

Information Overload

A state in which a team or individual receives more information than they can process meaningfully. This often leads to a paradoxical situation where, despite an abundance of data, the quality of decisions decreases because it becomes difficult to distinguish essential from non-essential information.

Redundancy

Refers to the multiple presence of the same information in a group's communication system. While avoiding redundancy increases efficiency, a certain degree of targeted repetition can ensure comprehensibility and reduce the risk of misunderstandings in critical tasks.

Stakeholder

Refers to all individuals or groups that have a legitimate interest in the outcome of a group project or are affected by its decisions. Early identification of stakeholders is crucial to consider their requirements and minimize resistance during the project.

Efficiency of Communication Structures

Comparison of problem-solving efficiency in different team communication networks.

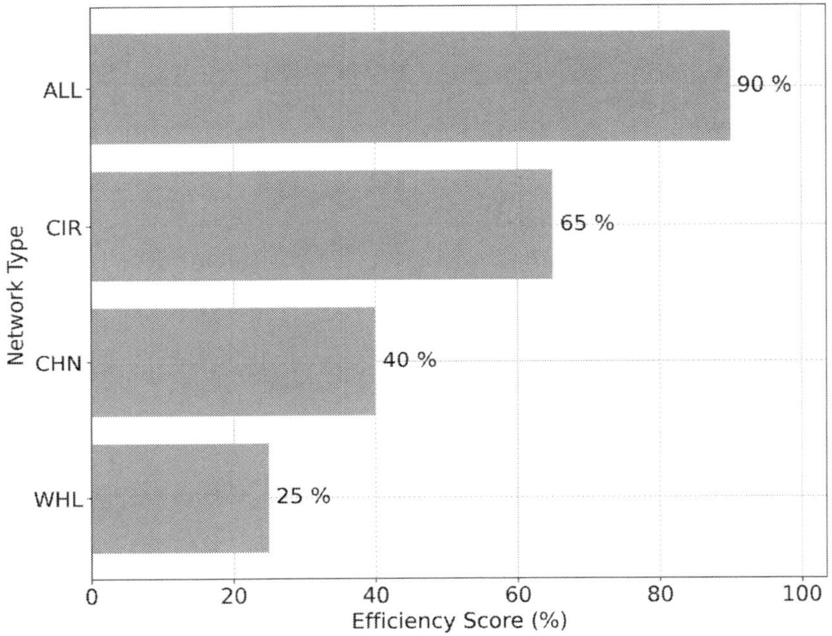

ALL: All-Channel (Decentralized)

CIR: Circle

CHN: Chain

WHL: Wheel (Centralized)

The chart illustrates how different communication structures impact a team's efficiency in solving complex problems. The fully connected (All-Channel) network, where every member can communicate directly with every other, is by far the most effective. This allows for a rapid exchange of ideas and feedback, fostering collaboration and innovation. In contrast, centralized structures like the 'Wheel' or linear ones like the 'Chain' create information bottlenecks and hinder the free flow of information, making them significantly less suitable for complex tasks that require diverse input. These values are estimations intended to demonstrate the fundamental principles of group dynamics. The key takeaway is that for complex challenges, decentralized and open communication channels are crucial for maximizing team performance.

3. 2 Effective Decision-Making Processes in Groups

Group decisions promise superior outcomes but often fail due to psychological pitfalls. Conformity pressure creates a false consensus, while discussions tend to gravitate towards extreme positions. Valuable contributions are lost in unstructured debates dominated by a few members. The root cause rarely lies in a lack of competence but rather in the uncontrolled dynamics of exchange. Therefore, the quality of a decision significantly depends on the design of the underlying process. This chapter presents practical methods to manage these dynamics and activate the full potential of the group for informed decisions.

The quality of a group decision depends less on spontaneous harmony or the persuasiveness of individual members than on the conscious establishment of processes that structure dissent and deliberately interrupt conformity pressure.

"

I shall assume that your silence gives consent.

"

Plato

Cratylus
435b

Plato's statement identifies a critical, and often dangerous, pitfall in group decision-making. The assumption that silence equals agreement can lead to 'groupthink' and false consensus, where individual doubts are suppressed in favor of perceived group harmony. Effective group processes require creating an environment where dissent is encouraged and silence is questioned, ensuring that decisions are based on genuine agreement rather than the absence of expressed opposition.

3.2.1 Measures for Preventing Groupthink

To prevent groupthink, several proven approaches exist that aim to modify leadership behavior, group structures, and communication norms. These methods are designed to ensure that decision-making processes are not compromised by the pressure to conform but are based on a broad and critical information base.

A central role is played by group leadership. Leaders can actively counteract groupthink by adopting a stance of Impartiality. They should refrain from expressing a preferred solution or opinion at the beginning of a discussion. When leadership reveals its position early on, group members tend to align their contributions with that guideline, whether out of respect, loyalty, or fear of negative consequences. Instead of steering the debate, leadership should promote an open and critical examination of all conceivable alternatives. This includes explicitly encouraging dissent and the expression of doubts. Leadership can institutionalize this culture of critical thinking by formally assigning a member to take on the role of critical challenger at each meeting.

Structuring the decision-making process itself provides effective levers to avoid conformity pressure. Instead of conducting all discussions in the plenary, the entire group can be divided into several smaller subgroups that work on the same problem in parallel. These subgroups initially develop their solutions independently. When the groups reconvene to present and discuss their results, a broader spectrum of perspectives emerges. The likelihood that all subgroups randomly arrive at the same, potentially flawed conclusion is low. This approach ensures that alternative viewpoints are generated and incorporated into the final decision-making.

Another procedural measure is the establishment of an "Advocatus Diaboli" (Devil's Advocate). One or more members are officially tasked with systematically questioning the arguments of the majority and specifically looking for weaknesses, risks, and overlooked disadvantages of the favored option. By formally assigning this role, dissent transforms from a potentially disruptive action into a constructive and expected contribution. This relieves the respective member from the social pressure that can otherwise accompany dissenting opinions and forces the group to justify and defend its position more robustly.

Shifting the focus from internal harmony to an overarching, objective goal is an effective strategy. This can be compared to the situation in medical teams, where the concentration on providing the best possible patient care helps to view differing professional opinions as valuable contributions to problem-solving rather than as disruptions to team spirit. Translated to other contexts, this means that a project team should focus on the quality of the end product or the fulfillment of customer requirements. When the common goal is clearly defined and binding for all, criticism of a proposal is no longer perceived as a personal attack on the author but as a constructive attempt to achieve the common goal in the best possible way. This creates psychological safety, a climate in which members feel free to express concerns without fearing negative social consequences.

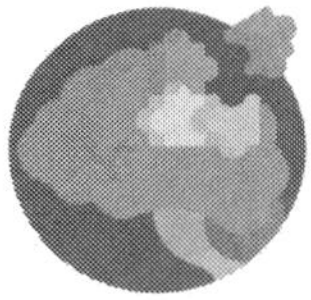

Additionally, seeking external feedback can break the internal perspective. Groups that work together for extended periods often develop a shared viewpoint and overlook information that does not fit their established schema. Deliberately consulting external experts or uninvolved colleagues can introduce new information and critical assessments into the process. These outsiders are not subject to the same group norms and loyalty dynamics and can therefore judge more impartially.

Finally, it is advisable to schedule a "second chance" meeting after a preliminary agreement. Between the two meetings, members should have time to reflect on the decision made and consider any lingering doubts. In the second meeting, these doubts are explicitly addressed. This time gap allows members to detach from the immediate social pressure of the first meeting and potentially revise their opinions without losing face. This ensures that the final decision withstands not only momentary consensus pressure but also subsequent critical scrutiny.

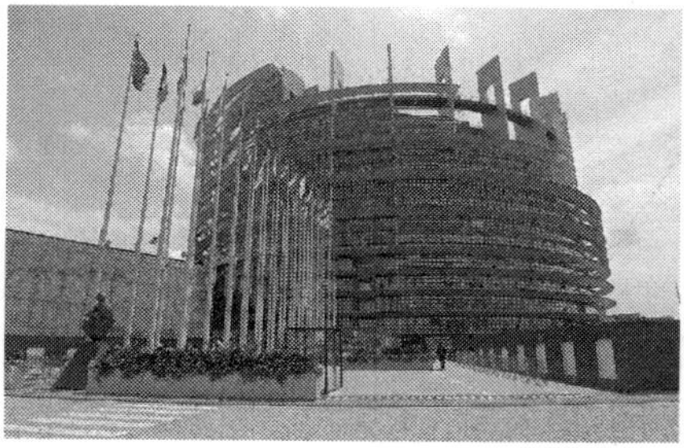

Plenum [i18]

Good to know

Advocatus Diaboli

A formally assigned role in which a group member is tasked with specifically finding counterarguments to a proposal and challenging the majority's position. This method makes dissent a legitimate part of the process and improves the quality of the argumentation.

Institutionalization

The embedding of certain processes or roles, such as that of the critical questioner, into the established rules of a group. This makes supportive behaviors a fixed part of the process and no longer dependent on the initiative of individual members.

Loyalty Dynamics

The functioning of personal bonds and commitments between group members. Such relationships can impair objective decision-making when agreement with a person becomes more important than the critical examination of their proposal.

Psychological Safety

A group climate in which members feel safe to express their opinions freely, ask questions, and admit mistakes without fearing negative social consequences such as exclusion or ridicule. It is the foundation for open communication and critical thinking.

Preventive Measures Against Groupthink

Conceptual weighting of different strategies for preventing groupthink.

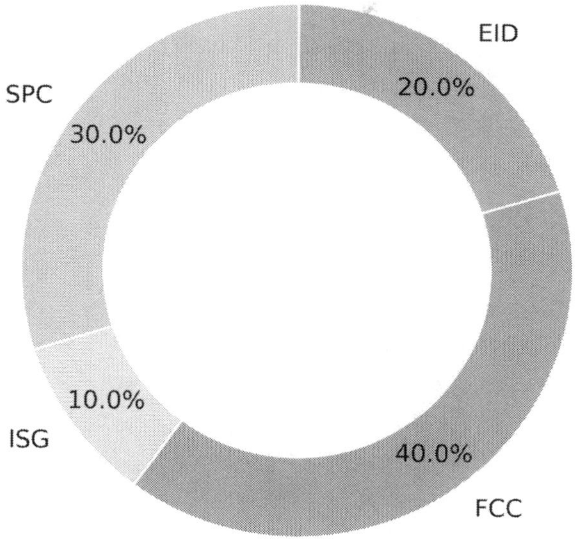

EID: External Input and Diversity

FCC: Fostering Critical Culture and Impartial Leadership

ISG: Individual Safeguards

SPC: Structural and Procedural Changes

The chart illustrates that fostering a culture of critical evaluation and ensuring impartial leadership is the most significant component (40%) in combating groupthink. This highlights the central role of the group's atmosphere and leadership style. Structural and procedural changes, such as appointing a 'devil's advocate' or breaking into subgroups, form the second most important pillar (30%). Actively seeking external input and ensuring diverse perspectives (20%) is crucial for breaking internal echo chambers. Finally, individual safeguards like anonymous feedback mechanisms (10%) provide an additional layer of protection. It is important to note that these figures are principled estimates intended to illustrate the relative importance of these categories. In practice, the optimal strategy is a combination of these measures, tailored to the specific context of the group and the decision.

3.2.2 Techniques for Mitigating Group Polarization

To counteract group polarization, which is the tendency of groups to adopt more extreme positions after a discussion than the original views of their members, targeted interventions in the communication and thinking process are necessary. These techniques aim to disrupt the two main drivers of polarization – the flow of one-sided arguments and social comparison pressure.

An effective approach lies in structuring the information exchange to prevent an avalanche of confirmation of a single perspective. In unmoderated discussions, members tend to express primarily those arguments they believe are shared by the majority. This creates a distorted picture of the actual distribution of opinions and reinforces the dominant viewpoint. One method to break this cycle is to consciously promote information diversity before an open debate begins. The group leader can ask all participants to first individually and in writing note the three strongest arguments for their position and additionally the strongest argument for the opposing position. These points are then presented in turn, without immediate evaluation or discussion. This procedure ensures that a wide range of arguments, including contradictory ones, is available from the outset, allowing the discussion to start on a more balanced foundation.

Another technique focuses on the deliberate search for disconfirming information to counteract the confirmation bias at the group level. Groups often reinforce their initial opinion because they focus on already known and shared information while ignoring facts that contradict that opinion. To prevent this, the task can be clearly defined to actively seek arguments and evidence that weaken the favored option. For example, a project team considering a new market entry can be tasked not only with analyzing the chances of success but also with conducting a detailed "pre-mortem" analysis. In this approach, the team imagines that the project has already failed and then systematically works backward to identify all conceivable reasons for this failure. This exercise forces the group to critically question their optimistic assumptions and engage with potential risks and negative aspects, thereby preventing a one-sided, risk-seeking polarization.

The mechanism of social comparison can also be directly addressed. Members often orient themselves to the perceived norms of the group and try to be a "good" member by representing a slightly sharper version of the group opinion. To mitigate this, moderation can explicitly change the norms of collaboration. Instead of rewarding conformity and determination, openness to changing opinions and the ability to integrate opposing viewpoints is established as the ideal. The group leader can model this value shift by publicly praising members who change their opinion based on compelling new arguments. This signals that the most valued position is not the most rigid but the most thoughtful and adaptable.

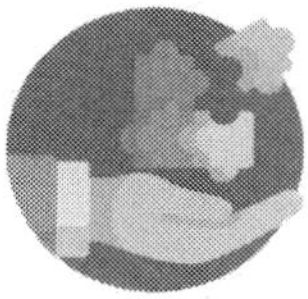

Finally, procedural interventions can help reduce the immediate social pressure that drives polarization. Utilizing anonymous voting or feedback systems at the beginning of a decision-making process can provide an unfiltered picture of the initial distribution of opinions before members influence each other. If a discussion still leads to a highly polarized stance, it is often advisable to postpone the final decision. A conscious "cooling-off period" of one or more days allows members to distance themselves from the emotional dynamics of the debate, rationally reconsider the arguments, and reassess their position without loss of face. This interruption weakens the urge to align with an extreme position out of social connectedness and promotes a more balanced final decision-making process.

Good to know

Confirmation Bias

Refers to the human tendency to preferentially seek and interpret information that supports one's existing opinion. In a group, this can lead to important counterarguments or risks being overlooked because they do not fit the favored solution.

Confirmation Bias

The internationally used technical term for confirmation bias. It describes the cognitive distortion that leads people to favor evidence that confirms their hypotheses while neglecting contradictory evidence.

Group Polarization

Describes the phenomenon where a group often makes a decision after a joint discussion that is more extreme than the average of the original individual opinions. This can lead to both riskier and more cautious outcomes, depending on the direction initially preferred by the group.

Pre-Mortem Analysis

A method of prospective thinking where a team imagines that a project has already failed. This retrospective thinking helps uncover potential weaknesses and risks that often remain undetected in purely optimistic planning.

Effectiveness of Mitigation Techniques on Group Polarization

Comparison of different techniques and their effect on reducing the degree of group polarization.

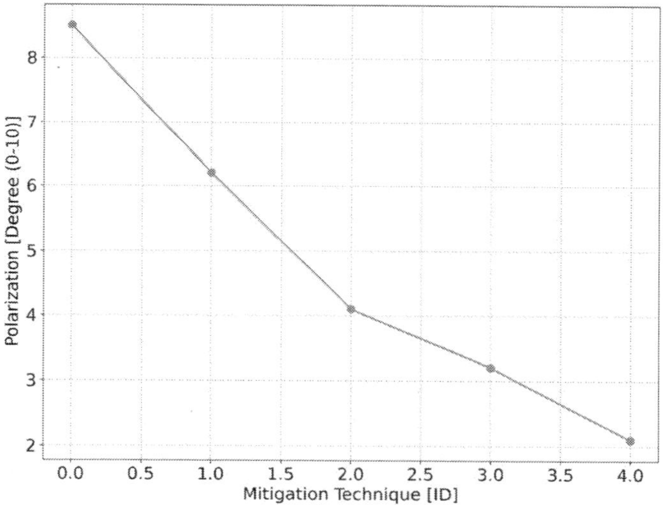

The chart illustrates the hypothetical effectiveness of various techniques in mitigating group polarization, where a higher value on the y-axis signifies a more extreme group opinion. The 'Control Group' (ID 0) establishes a baseline, showing a high degree of polarization in the absence of any intervention. A general instruction to 'Encourage Critical Evaluation' (ID 1) yields a moderate reduction. More structured and active interventions prove significantly more effective: Appointing a 'Devil's Advocate' (ID 2) to challenge the consensus and actively 'Introducing Diverse Perspectives' (ID 3) both lead to a substantial decrease in polarization. The most effective method shown is a 'Structured Discussion' format (ID 4), such as the Nominal Group Technique, which minimizes conformity pressure and results in the lowest level of polarization. It is important to note that these values are principled estimations intended to visually represent the general findings in social psychology research; they do not stem from a single, specific study.

3.2.3 Implementation of Effective Moderation Methods

The implementation of effective moderation methods shifts the focus from unstructured debates to a deliberately designed communication process. A moderator does not act as a content decision-maker but as an architect of the conversation flow. Their task is to create the conditions under which a group can unleash its full potential for problem-solving. This begins with establishing a clear agenda and transparent rules of engagement that are comprehensible to all members before the actual discussion starts. Such rules may limit speaking time, determine the order of contributions, or define how interruptions are handled to ensure that communication proceeds in an orderly and fair manner.

A central element of moderation is the active management of participation. In many groups, extroverted or high-ranking members dominate the discussion, while reserved or critical voices remain unheard. To counteract this imbalance, moderation employs structured techniques. Instead of an open round where the loudest voices prevail, a sequential inquiry of all opinions can take place. In this approach, all participants are asked in turn to briefly present their perspective on a topic before an open discussion begins. Another option is the method of silent brainstorming, where ideas are initially noted by each individual on cards. These cards are then collected, grouped visibly for all, and only then discussed together. Both approaches decouple idea generation from social pressure and ensure that contributions from otherwise quieter members are equally integrated into the process.

Moderation also ensures the focus and systematization of content. While discussions can easily go off track or get lost in details, the moderator keeps the thread intact. An effective tool for this is visualization. Key statements, arguments, open questions, and agreements already made are recorded visibly on a flip chart, whiteboard, or in a digital document for all to see. This shared visual reference creates transparency, prevents misunderstandings, and avoids the repetition of points already discussed. When the group begins to argue in circles, the moderator can refer to the visualization and steer the discussion toward the next logical step, for example, by asking: "We have summarized the arguments for A and B here. Which criterion helps us now in the evaluation?"

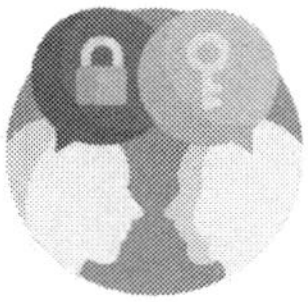

High-quality moderation transforms destructive conflict into constructive engagement. When two positions clash irreconcilably, the moderator intervenes to prevent escalation and reveal the underlying interests. An effective technique is to ask the opponents to summarize each other's position in their own words until the other confirms that their viewpoint has been correctly understood. Only then may their own response follow. This approach compels active listening and de-escalates the situation, as it transitions from pure confrontation to an attempt at mutual understanding. It can be compared to the work of a mediator, who does not dictate the solution but shapes the process so that the parties can find common ground themselves. The moderation also specifically protects those who express an unpopular opinion or criticism. It can explicitly recognize such contributions as valuable and remind the group that the task is to make the best decision, not the quickest or most harmonious one.

Finally, it is the moderator's responsibility to clearly define and guide the decision-making process itself. Before the final phase, it must be clarified how the decision will be made: Is the group aiming for a consensus, is a qualified majority sufficient, or is another procedure being followed? The moderator ensures that this procedure is accepted by all and guides the group through the final steps without influencing the outcome content-wise. Their neutrality regarding the result, while fully taking responsibility for the quality of the process, is key to gaining and maintaining the group's trust. Through this comprehensive design of the process, the likelihood of a well-founded decision supported by all members is maximized.

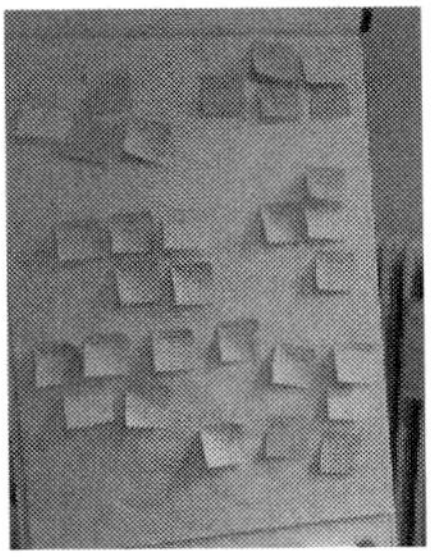

Silent Brainstorming [i19]

Good to know

Destructive Conflict

A form of confrontation where the factual debate is abandoned, and personal attacks, distrust, and the intent to harm the other take center stage. Such conflicts undermine cohesion and the group's ability to tackle future tasks.

Mediator

An impartial third party who mediates in a conflict without making a decision of their own. The main task is to restore communication between the disputing parties and help them recognize the underlying interests behind their positions.

Silent Brainstorming

A technique for idea generation where participants initially write down their thoughts individually and without verbal communication. This approach reduces the fear of direct evaluation by others and prevents dominant individuals from steering the first phase of idea generation.

Visualization

The recording of discussion content on a visible surface for all. This serves as a shared external memory for the group and relieves the cognitive resources of individual members. By objectifying ideas and arguments, they can be more easily separated from the individuals and evaluated more objectively.

Effectiveness of Group Decision-Making Methods

Decision quality by method structure and optimal group size.

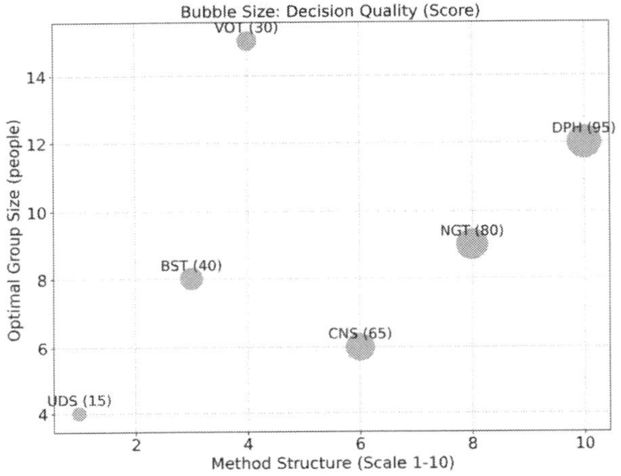

Blasengröße: Decision Quality (Score)

BST: Brainstorming

DPH: Delphi Method

UDS: Unstructured Discussion

CNS: Consensus Decision

NGT: Nominal Group Technique

VOT: Majority Vote

This chart illustrates how the quality of a group decision is influenced by the decision-making method used and the size of the group. The main takeaway is that more structured methods generally lead to higher-quality decisions (larger bubbles). Techniques like the Nominal Group Technique (NGT) and the Delphi Method excel because they systematically mitigate common group dysfunctions like 'groupthink', social loafing, and the dominance of a few voices. In contrast, less structured approaches like simple unstructured discussions or majority votes often yield lower-quality outcomes. The vertical axis shows that different methods are suited for different group sizes; for instance, achieving true consensus becomes exponentially harder in larger groups, whereas the Delphi Method can effectively handle larger, even anonymous, groups of experts. The data points are estimations intended to illustrate these fundamental principles of group psychology. The actual effectiveness of any method can vary depending on the specific context, the nature of the task, and the composition of the group.

3. 3 Conflict Management and Fostering Cohesion

In every group, different identities, goals, and opinions come together. This diversity is a strength, but it also carries the risk of conflict. Tensions between departments, the exclusion of outsiders, or suppressed dissent can paralyze collaboration, jeopardize success, and lead to stagnation. This chapter analyzes the psychological mechanisms behind these processes. It illuminates the path from competition to cooperation and the intentional building of cohesion. The focus is on constructively utilizing friction and integrating divergent perspectives as opportunities for better decisions and innovation. The following sections provide the tools to transform conflicts into productive energy and to shape teams into true performance units.

Sustainable conflict management does not eliminate differences but creates an overarching framework in which the diversity of perspectives and identities becomes a crucial resource for collective success.

> *When people are friends, they have no need of justice, but when they are just, they need friendship in addition.*

Aristotle

Nicomachean Ethics
Book VIII, 1155a.26

This quote perfectly illustrates the two pillars of a well-functioning group: social cohesion ('friendship') and clear processes ('justice'). Aristotle suggests that strong interpersonal bonds can often transcend the need for formal rules. However, in any group, formal fairness is essential, and it is most effective when complemented by positive relationships. This highlights the dual approach needed in conflict management: addressing the issue through fair processes while simultaneously working to strengthen the group's social fabric.

3.3.1 De-escalation of intergroup conflicts

The de-escalation of conflicts between groups fundamentally differs from the mediation of personal disputes. It requires an approach that analyzes the underlying group processes rather than merely the relationships of individual actors. At the core of these processes lies social identity. This arises from the feeling of belonging to a specific social group and profoundly influences how individuals perceive themselves and others. This identity can strengthen cohesion within one's own group (the "in-group") but often leads to the devaluation and distancing from other groups (the "out-groups"). Conflicts escalate when the boundaries between groups seem insurmountable and one's group identity is primarily defined by the distinction from the opponent.

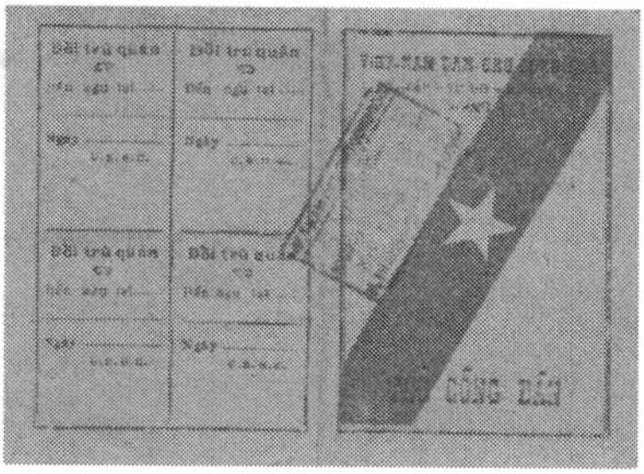

social identity [i20]

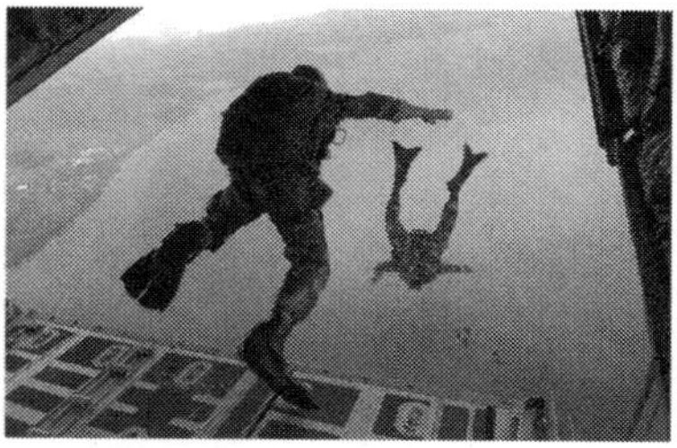

in-group [i21]

Structural conditions and the surrounding context can amplify these dynamics. When there are unequal power relations, unequal access to resources, or differing statuses between groups, this fosters a sense of injustice and heightens the perception of threat. Such structural inequalities often serve as the catalyst that transforms latent tensions into open conflicts. A change in context, such as a reorganization of departments in a company or new political legislation, can disrupt existing patterns of group interaction and contribute either to escalation or, if managed correctly, to de-escalation.

An effective approach to de-escalation is the conscious creation of a superordinate, shared identity that includes the previously opposing groups. The goal is not to erase the original group identities but to establish a new, more attractive "in-group" where the old group boundaries lose relevance. Members of the competing groups must recognize that they are part of a larger whole with common goals. This process succeeds when the superordinate identity is designed to acknowledge and appreciate the specific skills and contributions of the subgroups.

In a hospital where the departments of surgery and anesthesia frequently dispute resources and responsibilities, a purely mediating approach may fail as it ignores the deeply rooted professional identities. A de-escalating strategy here would be the establishment of an interdisciplinary "Patient Safety Team" that pursues a common and undeniably positive goal. In this new framework, the participants are no longer primarily surgeons or anesthetists working against each other but members of an expert team collaborating. The specific expertise of each group is needed to achieve the overarching goal and is thus elevated rather than serving as a point of competition. Mobilizing such a shared identity can foster collaboration and contribute to de-escalation [s18].

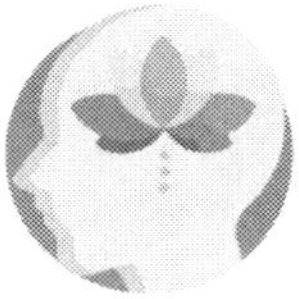

Implementing such changes requires careful planning, as any attempt to alter identities may encounter resistance if perceived as a threat to the existing group. It is therefore essential to actively involve the members of the involved groups in the process and to clearly communicate the benefits of the new, shared identity. Concrete measures to promote a superordinate identity include:

- Defining common goals that can only be achieved through cooperation and that provide clear benefits for all involved.
- Designing communication and workflows to actively promote and reward exchange and collaboration across the old group boundaries.
- Celebrating successes visibly that have been achieved through the cooperation of the new, larger team to link the positive experience with the superordinate identity.

In this way, the focus shifts from the divisive characteristics of the past to a shared, constructive future. De-escalation occurs not by ignoring or suppressing group identities but by purposefully evolving them towards a more inclusive and cooperative form of cohesion.

Good to know

Cooperation

Describes a form of social interaction in which two or more individuals or groups work together to achieve common benefits. It stands in contrast to competition, where the success of one party often means the failure of another.

De-escalation

Refers to targeted measures to reduce the intensity and hostility in a conflict. Instead of allowing a confrontation to escalate, specific communication techniques and structural changes are utilized to transition the involved parties into a more constructive state.

Out-group

Refers to a social group to which an individual does not feel they belong. These groups are often perceived as more homogeneous than one's own group and can become targets of negative stereotypes or prejudices.

Social Identity

This term describes the part of a person's self-concept that derives from membership in a social group. This sense of belonging is often associated with emotional significance and appreciation that accompanies this membership.

Effectiveness of De-escalation Tactics

Estimated success rates of different strategies in resolving intergroup conflicts.

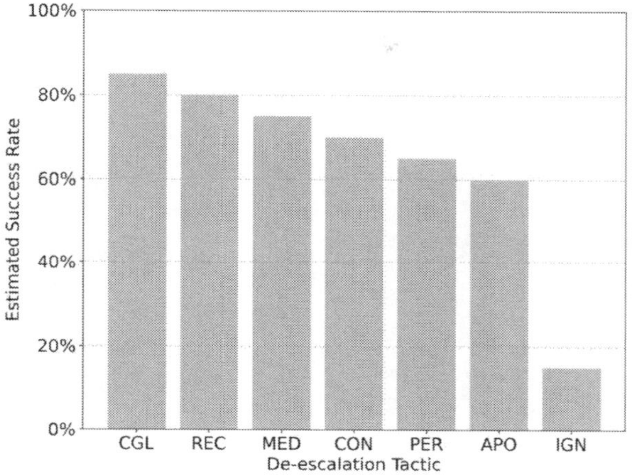

APO: Apology and Forgiveness
CON: Positive Intergroup Contact
MED: Mediation / Negotiation
REC: Recategorization (We-Identity)
CGL: Finding Common Goals
IGN: Ignoring the Conflict
PER: Perspective-Taking

The success rates presented are estimations based on established social psychological principles and models, intended to illustrate the fundamental effectiveness of various approaches. It is evident that collaborative and empathy-based tactics, which focus on creating shared identities or objectives, show the highest potential for success. Strategies like 'Finding Common Goals' and 'Recategorization' are particularly effective because they restructure the conflict from an 'us vs. them' dynamic to a 'we' perspective. Communicative approaches such as 'Mediation' and 'Perspective-Taking' also prove highly effective by fostering mutual understanding and dismantling stereotypes. In stark contrast, 'Ignoring the Conflict' is shown to be a highly ineffective strategy. While it may offer temporary relief, it fails to address the underlying issues, which often leads to the conflict festering and intensifying over time. The key takeaway is that active, integrative, and empathetic strategies are significantly superior to passive or avoidant behaviors for achieving lasting de-escalation and promoting group cohesion.

3.3.2 Strengthening Group Cohesion Through Common Goals

Common goals serve as a mechanism to solidify group cohesion. However, the effect does not arise solely from the mere existence of an initiative. The effectiveness of the goal as a binding element depends on its specific design and the manner in which it is communicated and pursued. A goal fosters cohesion most effectively when it is perceived by group members as desirable and simultaneously achievable. The perceived importance imbues the collective action with a sense that transcends individual task fulfillment, creating a shared motivation. At the same time, the assessment of attainability protects the group from demotivation and frustration that can arise from seemingly unattainable objectives. A leader can actively shape this perception by conveying not only the end result but also the value of the journey toward it. Thus, the abstract goal of completing software transforms into the tangible and meaningful endeavor of creating a tool that simplifies work processes for hundreds of colleagues. This communicated higher purpose enhances the personal attachment of members to the group goal [s19].

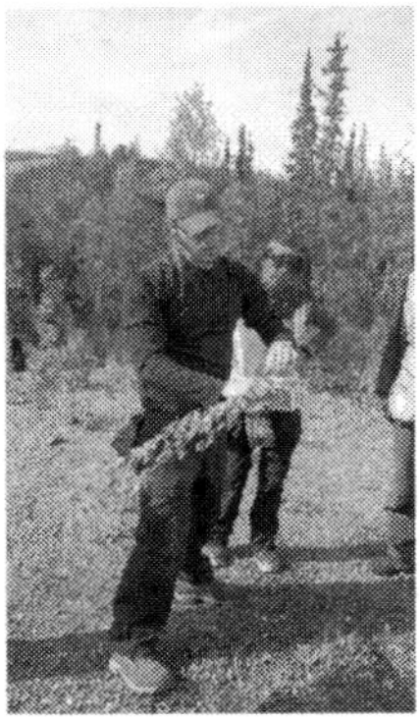

Identification [i22]

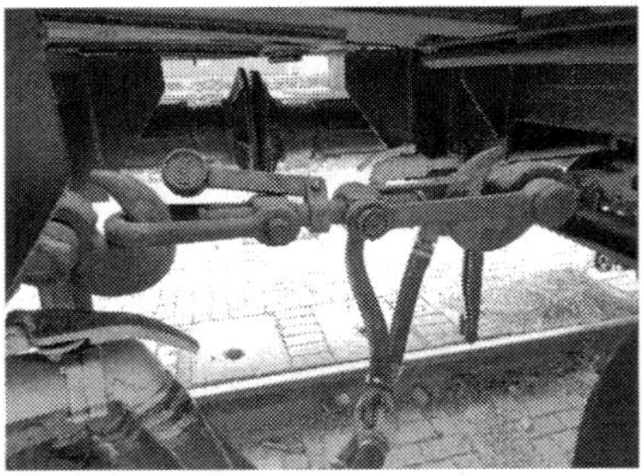

Interdependence [i23]

The process of pursuing goals itself acts as a social adhesive. An optimally formulated goal requires interdependence, meaning that members rely on one another for success. The contributions of individual members must interlock, inevitably leading to more intense exchange and closer coordination. In this phase of collaboration, initial differences among individuals fade into the background. Instead, members discover functional commonalities: a similar work ethic, complementary skills, or shared problem-solving competencies. This experience of pulling together despite all differences and being able to rely on one another is a strong driver of cohesion. The group perceives itself as a functioning unit, nurturing a sense of belonging and mutual trust. The identification shifts from the individual to the collective; the success of the group becomes a personal success [s20].

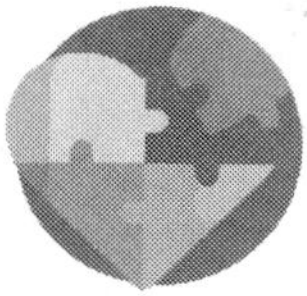

Continuous communication about progress and the adjustment of strategy are necessary to maintain momentum. Regular, transparent updates on achieved milestones make progress visible and reinforce the belief that the goal can be reached. This is particularly relevant when the path to the goal is long. Acknowledging partial successes creates positive, shared experiences that solidify the commitment of all involved. A project leader who is not solely fixated on the end date but consciously creates space to reflect together on the successful completion of a complex phase strengthens the collective efficacy expectation. Members see that their efforts bear fruit, which increases motivation for the next steps. Observing the engagement of other members can also be contagious and initiate a positive cycle of willingness to perform [s20].

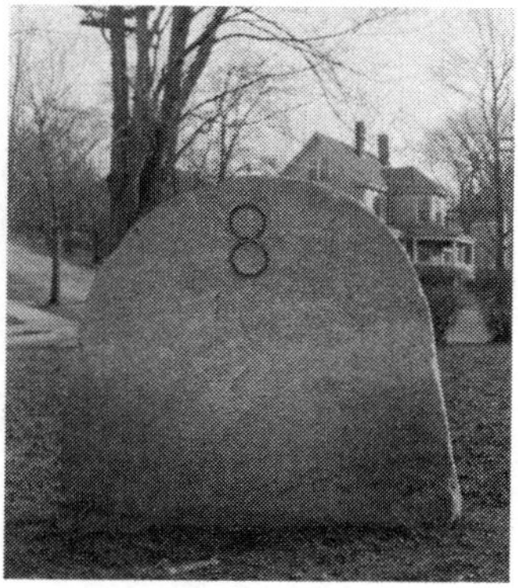

milestone [i24]

The social fabric of the group is further strengthened by interactions that go beyond purely task-related collaboration. While the formal structure of collaboration is dictated by the common goal, cohesion often solidifies in informal moments. A team that undertakes a charitable project, such as establishing a community garden, pursues not only the goal of planting and maintaining beds. During breaks, while engaging in physical work together, or while planning the next steps, conversations and relationships emerge that reach a deeper personal level. These informal contacts build a robust social network that supports the group even in times of disagreement or setbacks. The shared work on a tangible goal, combined with space for informal exchange, creates an environment where professional cooperation and personal connection mutually reinforce each other. Thus, the path to the goal—the sum of shared efforts, collective problem-solving, and experienced progress—shapes and unites the group.

Good to know

Collective Efficacy Expectation

The shared belief of a group that they can successfully perform the necessary actions to achieve specific goals together. A high expectation influences the choice of goals, the effort expended, and perseverance in the face of difficulties.

Group Cohesion

Refers to the strength of the bond and sense of 'we' within a group. It consists of the mutual attraction of members and the shared commitment to the group task. High cohesion can enhance willingness to perform but also carries the risk of suppressing dissenting opinions.

Identification

The process by which an individual perceives belonging to a group as an important part of their own self-definition. This leads to the group's successes and failures being experienced as one's own and can result in a preference for one's own group over others.

Interdependence

Describes the mutual dependence of individuals in a group. There is a distinction between task interdependence, where members depend on each other to complete their work, and outcome interdependence, where rewards or consequences apply to the entire group.

Goal Clarity and Group Cohesion

This chart shows the positive correlation between the clarity of a group's goals and its level of social cohesion.

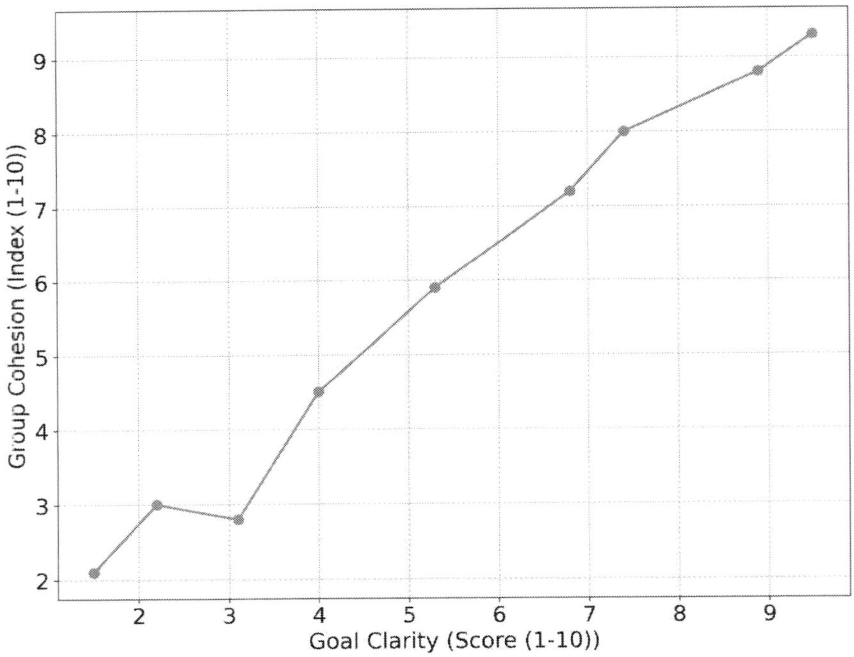

The data clearly indicates a strong positive relationship between goal clarity and group cohesion. Groups with vague, poorly defined goals (low values on the x-axis) tend to exhibit low levels of cohesion, often marked by internal friction and a lack of unified effort. As goals become more specific, measurable, and shared among members (higher values on the x-axis), the group's cohesion (y-axis) increases significantly. This suggests that clear objectives are a foundational element for building a strong team. They align members' actions, provide a common purpose, reduce conflicts over the group's direction, and foster a shared identity, ultimately leading to greater collaboration and mutual support.

3.3.3 The Integrative Approach to Outsiders and Deviating Opinions

The integrative approach to outsiders and deviating opinions

Groups develop a natural pressure for conformity aimed at maintaining harmony and agreement. This pressure often targets individuals whose views deviate from the consensus of the majority or who are perceived as outsiders. The group's reaction to such deviations is an indicator of its maturity and capacity for development. A group that suppresses dissent risks cognitive stagnation and flawed decisions, a phenomenon known as groupthink. In such an environment, agreement with the status quo is rewarded, while critical objections are seen as disloyal disruptions. This creates a burdensome situation for the deviating member: the desire for belonging conflicts with personal conviction, potentially leading to social withdrawal or reluctant conformity. In both cases, the group loses a valuable resource.

Deviating opinions are highly beneficial for the quality of group decisions. They compel the majority to reconsider their position, sharpen arguments, and explore alternatives that would otherwise remain unexamined. A single member advocating a counter-position can break the cognitive inertia of the group and initiate a deeper processing of information. Even if the deviating opinion ultimately proves incorrect, it has served its purpose by placing the final decision on a more solid, well-considered foundation. Thus, the role of the dissident is not one of division, but of quality assurance. The same applies to newcomers who join a group. Their unbiased perspective from the outside can reveal entrenched routines and blind spots that have long become invisible to long-standing members. Their integration thus represents an opportunity to foster the group's self-reflection and stimulate innovation.

Constructively managing these dynamics requires a proactive shaping of group culture, which can be actively promoted by a leader or the group members themselves. Instead of isolating dissenting voices, structures must be created that recognize and channel their contributions. For instance, a facilitator in a meeting where a unified opinion quickly forms can specifically address those members who have held back and explicitly ask them to identify potential weaknesses or alternative solutions. This act signals to the entire group that differing perspectives are not only tolerated but welcomed. This increases psychological safety—the conviction that one can express opinions and raise concerns without fear of negative consequences for one's reputation or career.

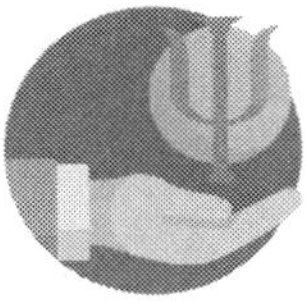

To establish such a culture, groups can agree on explicit behavioral norms that govern the handling of disagreements. These norms shift the focus from the person to the substantive level and de-emotionalize the discourse.

- Criticism is always directed at ideas and proposals, never at the person expressing them.
- Arguments are evaluated based on their validity, regardless of the status or popularity of the speaker.
- The role of the "Advocatus Diaboli" is institutionalized by assigning a member the task of actively seeking and presenting counterarguments during important decisions.

Such measures transform potential conflicts into a productive dialogue. Genuine group cohesion is not reflected in the absence of disagreements but in the group's ability to endure, process, and leverage them for its own goals. A group that learns to integrate its outsiders and contrarians is not only fairer but also more adaptable, innovative, and ultimately more successful in pursuing its common objectives.

Good to know

Advocatus Diaboli

A deliberately assigned role in a group tasked with consciously finding and presenting counterarguments to a prevailing opinion or proposal. The method is particularly effective when the role is taken seriously and not merely understood as a symbolic exercise.

Cognitive Stagnation

Describes a state in which a group stops developing new ideas or critically questioning existing assumptions. This stagnation often occurs in very homogeneous groups or when a lack of new stimuli and a fear of failure hinder creativity.

De-emotionalization

A process aimed at removing emotional charge from a discussion or conflict. This often occurs through the application of fixed conversation rules or a focus on factual information to enable a solution-oriented and rational engagement.

Psychological Safety

Refers to the shared belief among team members that it is safe to take interpersonal risks. In such an environment, individuals feel free to admit mistakes, ask questions, and contribute ideas, which is a fundamental basis for learning processes and high performance.

Distribution of Efforts in Integrative Conflict Management

Distribution of efforts for the successful integration of outsiders and dissenting opinions within a group.

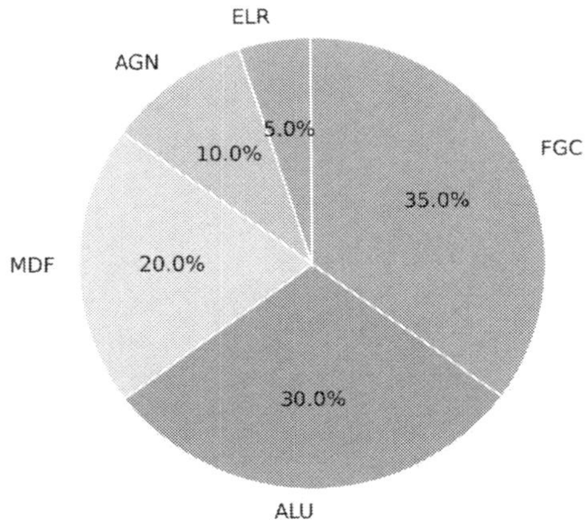

AGN: Adapting Group Norms and Processes

ALU: Active Listening and Understanding

ELR: Emotional Labor and Relationship Building

FGC: Finding Common Ground and Compromise

MDF: Mediation and Facilitation

The chart illustrates a hypothetical distribution of efforts in the complex process of integrating outsiders. These figures are estimates intended to depict the general principles and relative importance of the various activities. The largest share, 'Finding Common Ground and Compromise' (35%), highlights that the core of successful integration lies not just in discussion, but in the active, often arduous, work of building bridges and negotiating solutions. 'Active Listening and Understanding' (30%) is also a major component, emphasizing that genuine integration cannot occur without a deep and empathetic understanding of the divergent perspective. 'Mediation and Facilitation' (20%) represents the structured effort needed to guide these sensitive processes productively. The smaller but crucial segments, 'Adapting Group Norms' (10%) and 'Emotional Labor' (5%) underscore that integration is a holistic process that requires both structural flexibility from the group and sustained emotional investment from its members.

Concrete Advice

- Form targeted tandem partnerships between members of opposing groups who must collaboratively solve a third, neutral task to create personal relationships beyond group boundaries.
- Create a shared timeline where all subgroups can record their key past successes and challenges to foster mutual respect for each other's history.
- Establish a regular 'Workshop of Open Questions' where each member can present a current problem for which they cannot find a solution alone, institutionalizing a willingness to help.
- Define a physical 'Conflict Table' as the only permitted place for contentious debates, consciously ritualizing disputes and decoupling them from the everyday workplace.
- Have the group develop a shared metaphor for their ideal collaboration, such as 'Research Expedition' instead of 'Rowing Galley,' to shape a common understanding.
- Conduct a 'Success Autopsy' before a challenging endeavor, where you envision the perfect conclusion and retrospectively identify the conflicts that had to be overcome to achieve it.
- Alternately assign the role of 'Host' for joint meetings to opposing departments, responsible for fair and structured conversation management.
- Establish a 'Resource Exchange' where teams can offer and request small support services, such as an hour of expert advice or the use of a device, transforming competition into cooperation.
- Begin sensitive discussions with a silent round, where each person anonymously writes down their main point, initially separating the arguments from the individuals.

Review - 3. Group Psychology in Practice: Shaping Dynamics and Collaboration

Translating the insights of group psychology into practice means becoming the invisible architect of collaboration. Instead of leaving group processes to chance, you consciously create an environment where human potentials are not merely added but multiplied. The starting point often lies in overcoming the inertia that sets in when responsibility diffuses within the collective. Rather than simply distributing tasks, you should establish clearly defined "responsibility spaces." This goes beyond mere identification; it grants each member the status of an expert in their area, whose contribution is not only visible but essential for the success of the whole. Imagine you are leading a large project: instead of breaking it down into 20 small, equal work packages, you could form four powerful "squads," each fully responsible for a critical milestone. These smaller units develop their own dynamics, stronger cohesion, and a culture of mutual commitment that deprives social loafing of its breeding ground.

However, the real art begins where individual contributions merge into an intelligent overall performance. This requires a carefully calibrated interaction architecture. A common mistake is the assumption that an open forum automatically leads to the best ideas. In reality, it often fosters the dominance of a few voices and the silence of the majority. Therefore, implement a dynamic communication control: use phases of silence for idea generation, during which everyone writes down their thoughts uninfluenced. Only afterward should you open the discussion. This secures cognitive diversity before social conformity pressure sets in. To prevent the danger of groupthink, establish a culture of productive dissent. An extremely effective method is the "pre-mortem analysis": ask your team to imagine that the project has already failed catastrophically. Together, all conceivable reasons for this failure are then collected. This shift in perspective depersonalizes criticism, turns the search for weaknesses into a creative act, and strengthens the final decision without jeopardizing psychological safety.

Every collaboration inevitably encounters friction, whether through disagreements or conflicts between established subgroups. Instead of viewing these as disturbances, you should perceive them as a valuable source of energy that needs to be channeled. When two departments, such as marketing and development, are caught in conflict, appeals to reason often fail against entrenched identities. The solution lies in creating a tangible, overarching goal that can only be achieved together. Form a small, temporary team from members of both camps tasked with solving a specific customer problem within two weeks. This shared focus on an external "opponent" – the customer's problem – transforms internal rivalry into external cooperation. A similar attitude is crucial when dealing with dissenting opinions. Do not view persistent dissent as a sign of disloyalty, but as an early warning system for the health of your group. If everyone immediately agrees in important discussions, this should be a red flag. Your role as a leader or moderator is then to actively seek out the quiet voices and protect critical remarks by saying, "That's an important point we haven't considered yet. Let's explore that."

Ultimately, designing successful teamwork is not a one-time act but a continuous process of cultivation. It resembles the work of a gardener who prepares the soil, ensures the right mix of plants, regularly waters, and weeds so that the whole can grow and thrive. The tools of social psychology provide you with a well-stocked toolbox for this purpose. The conscious and situationally adapted application of these methods transforms groups from mere working communities into learning, resilient, and highly synergistic systems. This requires courage, reflection, and the willingness to break established patterns, but the rewards – in the form of better results, higher motivation, and a more fulfilling collaboration – are worth the effort.

4. Interpersonal Relationships: Attraction, Conflicts, and Prosocial Behavior

Why are we spontaneously drawn to some people while others seem unlikable at first glance? The mechanisms that govern our social bonds follow psychological principles that extend far beyond first impressions. Whether we help others or reject them, how we resolve disagreements, and which factors promote lasting relationships—all of this can be explained by scientific insights. At the same time, research shows that seemingly irrational reactions, such as spontaneous antipathy or selfless behavior, follow understandable patterns. This chapter reveals the unconscious forces that guide our most important interpersonal decisions.

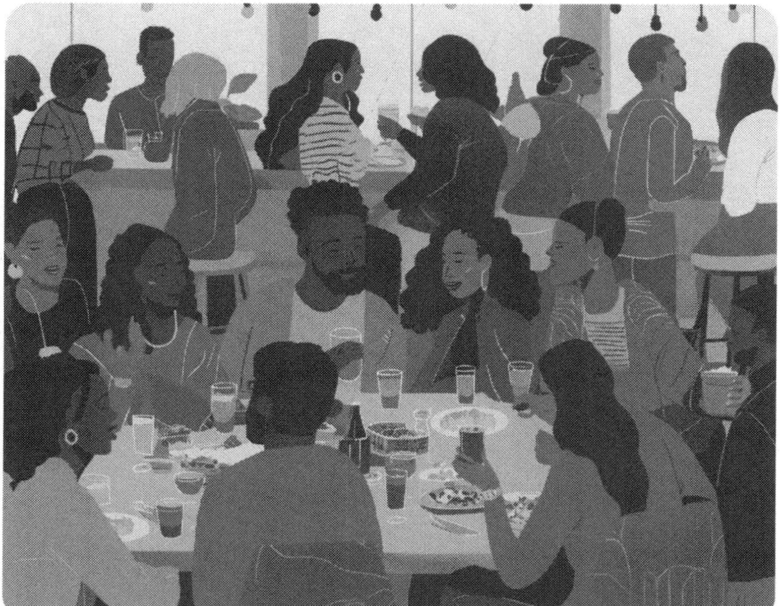

Prosociality and Conflict: A Historical Map

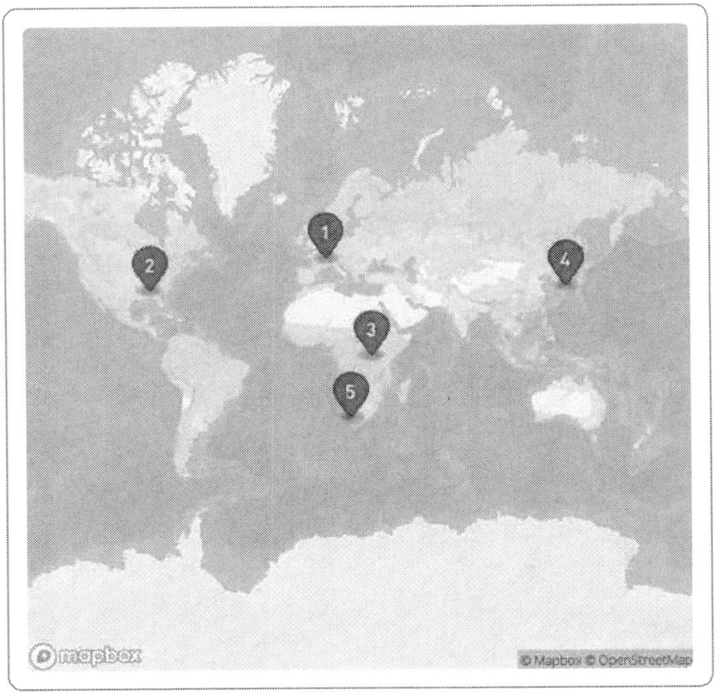

Key historical sites illustrating large-scale prosocial behavior (altruism, peace) and intergroup conflict (aggression).

1 **Geneva, Switzerland**

The birthplace of the Red Cross and the Geneva Conventions. This city symbolizes institutionalized altruism on a global scale. Following the horrors of war, the conventions established humanitarian laws, representing a collective prosocial effort to limit aggression and provide impartial aid, making the principles of humanitarianism attractive to nations worldwide.

2 **Selma, Alabama, USA**

A pivotal site of the American Civil Rights Movement. The 1965 Selma to Montgomery marches exemplify a clash between systemic aggression and non-violent protest. The marchers demonstrated profound altruism and attracted national support for the cause of racial equality, ultimately leading to the Voting Rights Act of 1965 and challenging entrenched intergroup conflict.

3 **Kigali, Rwanda**

The location of the Kigali Genocide Memorial, which commemorates the 1994 genocide against the Tutsi. This site is a stark reminder of the depths of intergroup aggression. In its aftermath, it has become a center for education and reconciliation, representing a difficult but essential prosocial effort to foster peace and prevent future atrocities through remembrance.

4 **Hiroshima, Japan**

The site of the first atomic bombing, an act of unprecedented aggression that ended World War II. In its wake, Hiroshima transformed into a global symbol of peace. The city's dedication to nuclear disarmament showcases a powerful shift from victimhood to advocacy, demonstrating a large-scale prosocial movement fueled by an attraction to a world free from nuclear weapons.

5 **Cape Town, South Africa**

The site of Robben Island, where Nelson Mandela was imprisoned, symbolizes the institutionalized aggression of Apartheid. Mandela's subsequent release and leadership of the Truth and Reconciliation Commission represents one of history's most significant examples of prosocial leadership, choosing altruistic reconciliation over retribution to heal a nation fractured by decades of intergroup conflict.

4. 1 Fundamentals of Social Attraction and Liking

Social attraction often appears random, yet it follows precise psychological patterns. Whether we form friendships or begin a partnership depends on unconscious processes that fundamentally shape our personal and professional lives. Understanding these mechanisms is crucial for building stable social networks and avoiding systematic misjudgments in assessing others. This chapter examines the most influential factors of sympathy. It highlights how the architecture of our daily lives, perceived similarities, and the first visual impression subtly guide our social judgments. Knowledge of these fundamentals allows us to comprehend the emergence of attraction and to consciously shape interpersonal relationships.

While chance and first impressions open the door to a new relationship, it is only shared values and a deep similarity of character that determine whether we enter and stay.

> *A noble person attracts noble people, and knows how to hold on to them.*

Johann Wolfgang von Goethe

Torquato Tasso, Act I, sc. i (1790)

Goethe's observation aligns closely with one of the fundamental principles of interpersonal attraction: the similarity-attraction effect. Social psychology has consistently shown that we are drawn to people who share our values, attitudes, and characteristics. The quote suggests that this attraction is not passive; 'nobility' (or shared qualities) actively draws like-minded individuals together and is key to maintaining those bonds over time.

4.1.1 The Importance of Proximity and Mere Exposure

Proximity is one of the simplest predictors of the formation of friendships and social bonds. People tend to build relationships with those they encounter most frequently in their daily lives. This relationship, known as the propinquity effect, was demonstrated in a classic study by Leon Festinger, Stanley Schachter, and Kurt Back in 1950 at a student dormitory at the Massachusetts Institute of Technology (MIT). The researchers found that the likelihood of friendship correlated directly with the distance between living units. The closest friendships were formed between next-door neighbors (41%), while the friendship rate decreased with increasing distance.

Even more revealing was the discovery of "functional distance." This refers not only to the physical distance in meters but also to the architectural design that influences the likelihood of casual encounters. Residents living near mailboxes, stairwells, or trash bins had disproportionately many friends throughout the building. They were positioned at junctions of daily life, providing more opportunities for contact with a larger number of housemates. This increased frequency of contact lays the groundwork for relationship building.

However, the increased likelihood of interactions alone does not explain the entire dynamic. Here, the mere exposure effect comes into play. This psychological phenomenon described by Robert Zajonc states that people tend to develop a preference for things simply because they are familiar. Repeated, neutral exposure to a stimulus—be it a face, a name, or a piece of art—leads to a more positive evaluation. Familiarity itself becomes a source of liking. Proximity ensures this repeated exposure. The face of a colleague at the next table, the person seen every morning on the train, or the neighbor who leaves the house at the same time become more familiar over time.

Thus, those seeking connection in a new social environment, such as at work or in a new city, can leverage these mechanisms. It is not about intrusive attempts at contact but rather about increasing one's visibility and the number of casual, neutral encounters. Specific behaviors that contribute to this include:

- Regular but unobtrusive presence in communal areas like the coffee kitchen or break rooms.
- Participation in shared, low-threshold activities such as lunch in the cafeteria or voluntary team events.
- Choosing a seat in the office or lecture hall that offers high visibility and proximity to pathways or central points.

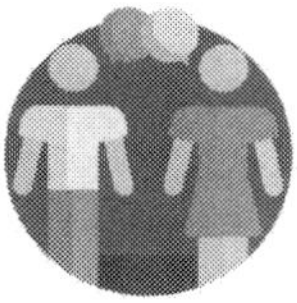

The psychological reasons for the effectiveness of mere exposure are multifaceted. On one hand, processing familiar stimuli requires less cognitive effort. This ease of processing (perceptual fluency) is often unconsciously and mistakenly interpreted as liking for the stimulus itself. On the other hand, familiarity signals safety and predictability. An unfamiliar face carries a residual risk, while a familiar person is perceived as less threatening and more predictable. Our brains prefer the familiar because it was evolutionarily advantageous to approach the unknown with caution.

However, the effect has limits and can reverse. If there is a negative attitude toward a person from the outset, repeated contact does not lead to liking but rather intensifies aversion. Each subsequent encounter confirms and solidifies the negative judgment. If the first interaction with a new colleague is unfriendly, their repeated presence is likely to increase the antipathy rather than decrease it. Similarly, an excessively high frequency of exposure can lead to saturation and boredom, diminishing the positive effect.

In summary, proximity creates the necessary opportunities for repeated, casual contacts. The mere exposure effect then ensures that this neutral familiarity can gradually evolve into liking, as long as the initial interactions are not negative. The architecture of our living and working spaces thus unconsciously shapes our social network.

Good to know

Mere Exposure Effect

A psychological principle stating that repeated, neutral exposure to a person or object leads to a more positive evaluation. This effect is deliberately used in advertising by frequently displaying logos and products to create familiarity and a positive baseline attitude in consumers.

Mere-Exposure Effect

The English term for the mere exposure effect. The effect occurs even when stimuli are presented subliminally, that is, unconsciously. This demonstrates how fundamental the processing of familiarity is for attitude formation.

Perceptual Fluency

Describes the ease with which a stimulus can be processed. This ease can relate not only to visual but also to auditory stimuli. For example, easily pronounceable names are often unconsciously rated as more likable and trustworthy.

Propinquity Effect

Refers to the phenomenon that proximity increases the likelihood of developing friendships and relationships. In the digital world, this effect can also arise from frequent virtual encounters in social networks or online games, understood as digital proximity.

Influence of Proximity and Exposure on Liking

Comparison of different social conditions on the development of interpersonal liking.

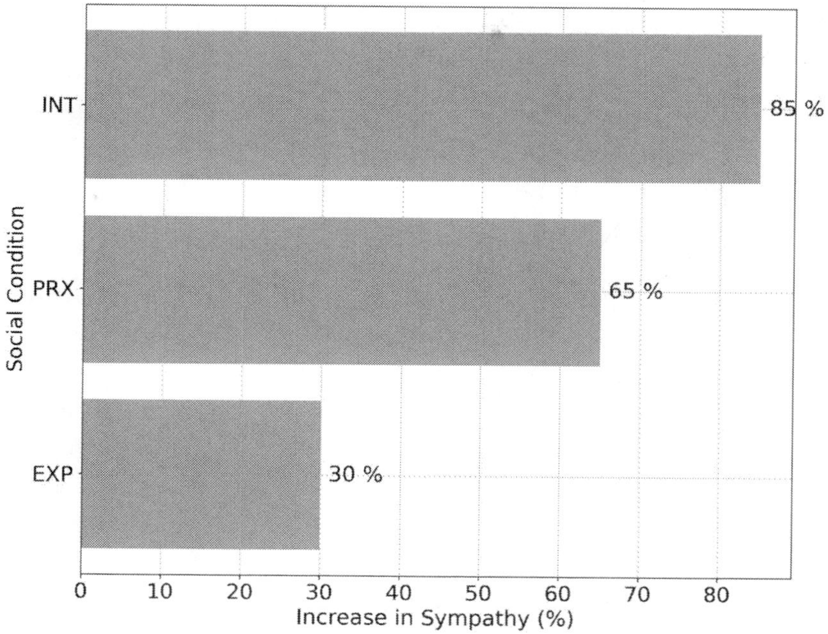

- EXP: Mere Exposure
- INT: Frequent Interaction
- PRX: Spatial Proximity

The chart illustrates the relative impact of mere exposure, spatial proximity, and active interaction on the formation of sympathy. Mere exposure to a person, without any interaction, already fosters a notable increase in liking. However, spatial proximity, which naturally increases the likelihood of unplanned, brief encounters, has a significantly stronger effect. The most substantial increase in sympathy occurs through frequent, meaningful interaction, which is often a direct result of sustained spatial proximity. These values are principled estimations designed to illustrate the fundamental mechanisms of social attraction as described in social psychology, rather than representing data from a single specific study.

4.1.2 Similarity as a Factor for Stable Relationships

After spatial proximity has created opportunities for encounters, another mechanism comes to the forefront that promotes the development of sympathy into a stable relationship: similarity. The saying "Birds of a feather flock together" summarizes a well-documented social psychological principle. People are attracted to individuals who are similar to them in various dimensions. These similarities are not random byproducts; rather, they serve multiple functions for relationship dynamics.

Attraction through similarity begins with easily observable demographic characteristics such as age, background, education level, and socioeconomic status. Such commonalities often create a shared experiential world and a similar frame of reference, facilitating initial communication. However, the alignment in attitudes, values, and beliefs runs much deeper. When we meet someone who shares our political views, ethical principles, or ideas of a successful life, we experience a social validation. The existence of another person who sees the world similarly to us reinforces our own, often deeply rooted beliefs. This generates a sense of correctness and belonging. In contrast, interaction with dissimilar individuals can trigger cognitive dissonance—a discomforting state that arises when our own views are challenged. The avoidance of this state unconsciously motivates us to turn to people who reflect our worldview rather than challenge it.

Moreover, similarity facilitates social interactions. Shared interests and hobbies provide an inexhaustible source for joint activities and conversation topics. Planning leisure time becomes easier when both partners enjoy similar activities, whether it be hiking, visiting museums, or following a particular sport. These smooth and positive interactions act as rewards, reinforcing mutual affection. We anticipate that future encounters with a similar person will also be pleasant and uncomplicated, which increases the motivation to maintain and deepen contact.

In the context of long-term partnerships, the similarity of personality traits gains particular relevance. While initial attraction is often sparked by shared interests, it is the matching personality profiles that can contribute to the stability of a relationship. Longitudinal studies suggest that the fit of certain character traits influences well-being in the partnership. A high degree of similarity in the personality trait "agreeableness"—the tendency to be cooperative, compassionate, and accommodating—correlates, for example, with higher relational well-being, especially among women, as it enhances perceived support in the relationship [s21]. A couple in which both partners exhibit high agreeableness is likely to resolve conflicts more cooperatively and constructively rather than falling into confrontational patterns.

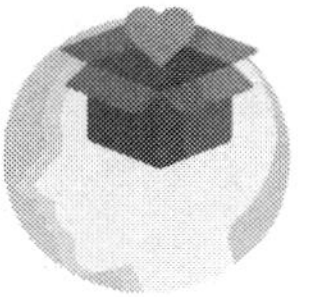

However, the dynamics are more complex than a simple formula stating that maximum similarity is always optimal. Research also shows that the specific combination of personality traits is crucial, not just the sheer agreement [s21]. In some areas, a certain degree of dissimilarity can even be advantageous and act as complementarity. A more introverted partner may benefit from the sociability of an extroverted partner, while the latter appreciates the calm and balance that the introverted partner provides. Here, dissimilarity does not become a source of conflict but rather a mutual enrichment, where one person's strengths compensate for the other's weaknesses.

For the conscious design of social relationships, it can be inferred to shift the focus. While superficial commonalities like the same taste in music are a good conversation starter, the search for agreement in fundamental values, life goals, and compatible personality traits proves to be more effective for the long-term stability of a bond. Self-reflection on one's non-negotiable core beliefs and traits is a first step in recognizing what type of similarity is necessary for one's well-being in a relationship.

Good to know

Complementarity

The principle that opposites attract because different traits or needs complement each other. A person seeks in another individual characteristics that compensate for their own weaknesses or fill a gap, which can lead to mutual enrichment.

Longitudinal Study

A research method in which the same individuals are repeatedly studied over an extended period. This allows for the observation and analysis of the development of relationships and changes in factors such as attitudes or satisfaction over time.

Social Validation

The need for confirmation of one's views and feelings by others. This validation strengthens self-esteem and the sense of belonging but can also lead to surrounding oneself primarily with like-minded individuals and avoiding divergent perspectives.

Similarity and Relationship Longevity

This chart illustrates the correlation between the degree of similarity and the average duration of a relationship.

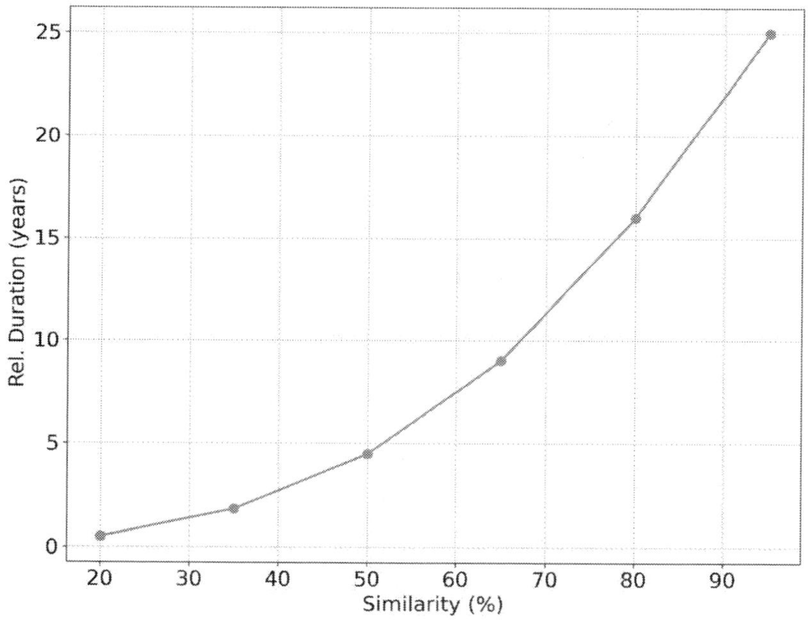

The data shows a clear positive correlation: the higher the measured degree of similarity between partners in core values and attitudes, the longer their relationship is projected to last. While relationships with low similarity (below 40%) show a significantly lower average duration, the longevity increases substantially with rising similarity. This suggests that shared foundations in beliefs, goals, and personality traits contribute significantly to reducing conflict and fostering long-term stability. A high degree of similarity acts as a strong predictor for a lasting partnership. It should be noted that these data are illustrative estimates designed to represent a fundamental principle of social psychology. They are not from a specific longitudinal study but serve to visualize the general, scientifically supported trend.

4.1.3 The Perception of Physical Attractiveness and Its Effects

Physical Attractiveness is a powerful factor in shaping social judgments and influences interpersonal attraction, with the gender of the individuals involved potentially modifying the strength of this effect [s22]. Our reaction to another person's appearance is often immediate and unconscious, even before a single word has been exchanged. This rapid assessment is based on a cognitive heuristic often described as "What is beautiful is also good." This is underpinned by the so-called Attractiveness Halo Effect: individuals whose faces are perceived as attractive are automatically attributed a range of other positive traits. Studies show that more attractive people tend to be rated as more sociable, competent, intelligent, and even healthier, without any objective evidence to support these claims [s23].

This unconscious bias has concrete consequences in social and professional contexts. In social and professional situations, it can lead to an unconscious preference. A candidate with a face deemed attractive may be unwittingly attributed higher social skills or better suitability for a customer-oriented position, even before their substantive qualifications are assessed. While this cognitive shortcut saves mental effort, it leads to systematic distortions in the evaluation of others.

The psychological causes of these strong effects are deeply rooted in our evolutionary past and the workings of our perception. One explanation is provided by the Hypothesis of Overgeneralized Face Perception. It posits that our brain extends adaptive responses, originally aimed at actual health or fitness traits, to purely external characteristics. A less attractive face is thus rated more negatively because it may exhibit features reminiscent of faces belonging to individuals with lower biological fitness, triggering instinctive caution [s23].

A specific mechanism in this context is the response to the Baby Schema. Faces with baby-like features—such as large, round eyes, a high forehead, and a small chin—trigger our care and protection instincts. Individuals with such traits are often perceived as more naive, warmer, honest, and submissive. Being aware of these mechanisms can sharpen one's self and other perception. This allows one to discern whether the assessment of a person—such as a colleague in a position of trust—is based on their actual behavior or unconsciously on their childlike facial features, which may be mistakenly interpreted as a guarantee of sincerity.

In addition to the static features of a face, fleeting emotional expressions also significantly influence our judgments. We tend to interpret a momentary facial expression as an indicator of a stable personality trait. A person who frequently smiles is perceived not only as currently happy but also as fundamentally friendlier and more approachable. Conversely, a neutral facial expression that appears grumpy or stern due to anatomy may be mistakenly interpreted as a sign of a hostile or aloof personality. Therefore, consciously managing one's facial expressions can actively shape social resonance. An open, friendly facial expression in new social situations, such as when greeting new team members, signals approachability and can lay the groundwork for positive subsequent interactions, regardless of the static features of the face. Understanding these unconscious processes enables one to critically question their first impressions and focus more on others' actual actions and communicated content, rather than being solely guided by appearances.

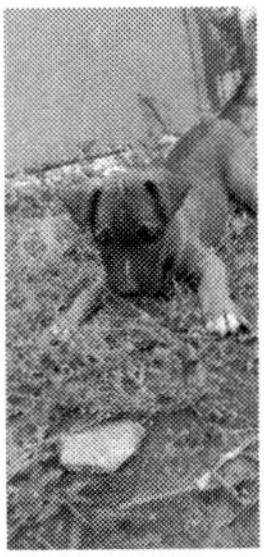

baby schema [i25]

Good to know

Attractiveness Halo Effect

A perceptual error where the positive trait of physical attractiveness radiates to other, independent personality domains. This effect often leads to attractive individuals being mistakenly attributed higher abilities or better character.

Biological Fitness

A measure of an individual's reproductive success compared to others. Traits indicating high biological fitness, such as health and strength, are often unconsciously perceived as attractive in mate selection.

Hypothesis of Overgeneralized Face Perception

The assumption that the human tendency to infer health and fitness from faces is applied excessively. Even slight deviations from an idealized face can lead to unjustifiably negative social judgments.

Physical Attractiveness

The evaluation of a person's external appearance, which may include culturally shaped beauty ideals and universal features such as facial symmetry. This evaluation significantly influences the first impression and the willingness to establish a social relationship.

Components of Physical Attractiveness Perception

Estimated contribution of various factors to the overall perception of physical attractiveness.

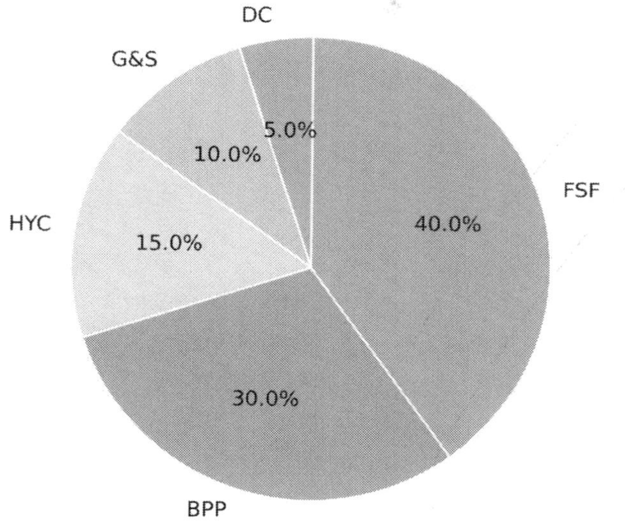

BPP: Body Proportions and Physique
FSF: Facial Symmetry and Features
HYC: Health and Youth Cues (Skin, Hair)
DC: Dynamic Cues (e.g., Smile, Posture)
G&S: Grooming and Style

The chart illustrates the estimated relative importance of different factors in the perception of physical attractiveness. It highlights that biological and evolutionary cues, such as facial features (40%) and body proportions (30%), are often the most significant contributors. These elements, like facial symmetry and the waist-to-hip ratio, are thought to signal genetic fitness and health. Health and youth cues, like clear skin and hair, further add to this perception (15%). However, factors that are more within an individual's control, such as grooming and personal style (10%), and dynamic cues like a confident posture or a warm smile (5%), also play a tangible role. It is important to note that these figures are estimations intended to illustrate the general principles of attractiveness perception, as the precise weighting can vary significantly based on cultural context, individual preferences, and the specific situation.

4. 2 Promoting Prosocial Behavior and Helpfulness

Prosocial behavior is a cornerstone of social interaction. Nevertheless, psychological barriers often hinder effective assistance. In emergencies, the bystander effect paralyzes individual initiative, while in everyday situations, the reluctance to ask for support blocks prosocial actions. This passivity undermines the stability of social relationships and individual well-being. This chapter therefore illuminates the psychological causes of omitted help and demonstrates how prosocial behavior can be deliberately promoted. It analyzes the mechanisms behind the bystander effect as well as the crucial roles of empathy, social norms, and the ability to ask for and accept help. The approaches presented here provide concrete tools to transform passive observation into active engagement.

Effective willingness to help is not a passive trait, but a learned social competence that equally encompasses the courageous intervention for others and the ability to ask for help oneself.

> *Noble be man, Helpful and good!*
> *For that alone Sets him apart From*
> *every other creature On earth.*

Johann Wolfgang von Goethe

Das Göttliche (The Divine) (1783)

This excerpt from Goethe's poem serves as an eloquent call to action for prosocial behavior. It frames helpfulness and goodness not merely as positive traits, but as the defining characteristic of humanity. In social psychology, the study of altruism and helping behavior explores why people engage in such acts. Goethe's verse provides a philosophical and moral foundation, suggesting that this capacity is a core part of what makes us human.

4.2.1 Action Steps to Overcome the Bystander Effect

To overcome the bystander effect, a multi-step process is required, beginning with the perception of the situation and culminating in targeted action. The mere presence of others can paralyze individual willingness to help, a phenomenon known as diffusion of responsibility. In this case, the individual observer assumes that another person will take responsibility and intervene. The first action step is to consciously break this psychological trap. Instead of distributing responsibility to an anonymous crowd, the individual must define the situation for themselves as an emergency and accept personal responsibility for intervening. This cognitive shift from a passive to an active role is the foundation for any further assistance. The likelihood that someone will help decreases with the number of bystanders present, as the perceived personal responsibility diminishes [s24]. Actively taking responsibility directly neutralizes this effect.

Another factor that significantly influences intervention is the social relationship between those involved. People are far more willing to intervene for friends, acquaintances, or even loosely connected individuals than for complete strangers. The existence of a social bond creates a sense of obligation and connection that can outweigh the inhibiting effect of others' presence [s24]. This insight can be practically utilized, even when there is no prior relationship with the victim. An effective strategy is to dissolve the anonymity of the group and create a temporary social unit. Instead of silently hoping that someone will act, a person can directly address other attendees and enlist them as allies. A clear request such as, "We need to do something. Can you help me call the ambulance while I take care of the person?" transforms passive bystanders into active helpers. This action not only delegates specific tasks but also creates a common goal and social support, lowering the threshold for all involved.

Once the decision to act has been made, the type of intervention matters. The belief in one's ability to positively influence a situation—the so-called self-efficacy—is a driver for successful intervention. This self-efficacy is strengthened when one has a repertoire of concrete action strategies. Programs promoting prosocial behavior show that verbal interventions, in particular, can be very effective in de-escalating or interrupting a situation without putting oneself in great danger [s25]. Such verbal expressions can be trained and applied situationally. They range from direct to indirect methods:

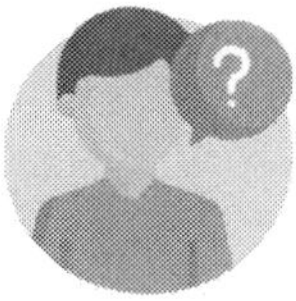

- **Direct Address**: Clearly and unequivocally instructing the aggressor to stop ("Leave the person alone!").
- **Distraction**: Asking an unexpected question or performing an action that diverts attention from the victim and interrupts the situation ("Excuse me, can you tell me how to get to the train station?").
- **Delegation**: Specifically asking other individuals for help and assigning them concrete tasks ("You in the blue coat, please call the police!").
- **Moral Appeal**: Referring to ethical norms or the wishes of the victim. Phrasing that targets the preferences of the affected person or general moral principles is particularly effective in influencing the aggressor's behavior ("This person doesn't want that.", "You shouldn't do that.") [s25].

The conscious application of these verbal techniques reduces uncertainty about what to do and increases the likelihood of a successful and safe intervention. They allow one to control the situation without necessarily having to engage in physical confrontation. The combination of taking personal responsibility, activating social dynamics, and employing learned, effective intervention strategies forms a comprehensive approach to breaking the passivity of the bystander effect and promoting prosocial behavior.

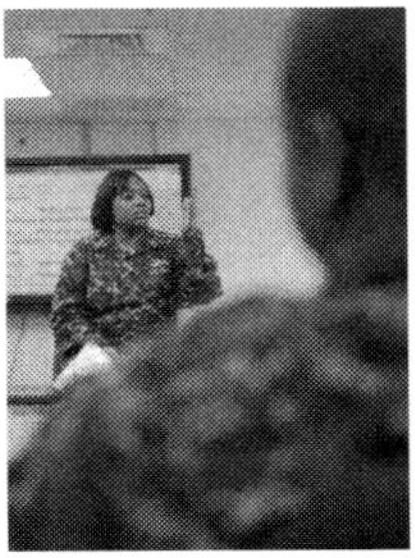

Intervention [i26]

Good to know

Bystander Effect

Refers to the phenomenon where the willingness to help in an emergency situation decreases with the increasing number of bystanders present. One reason for this is that individuals interpret the inaction of others as a sign that the situation is not serious and does not require intervention.

Diffusion of Responsibility

The process by which personal responsibility for necessary intervention is distributed among all present. This leads to no single person feeling responsible, thereby decreasing the overall likelihood of assistance.

Moral Appeal

A verbal strategy that appeals to conscience or recognized societal values to influence a person's behavior. The goal is to de-escalate a situation or mobilize help by referencing universally accepted ethical principles.

Self-Efficacy

The subjective belief of a person in their ability to successfully cope with a challenging situation on their own. In the context of helping, this is the belief that one's actions can make a positive difference.

Effectiveness of Interventions Against the Bystander Effect

Estimated likelihood of a person in need receiving help, based on different intervention strategies.

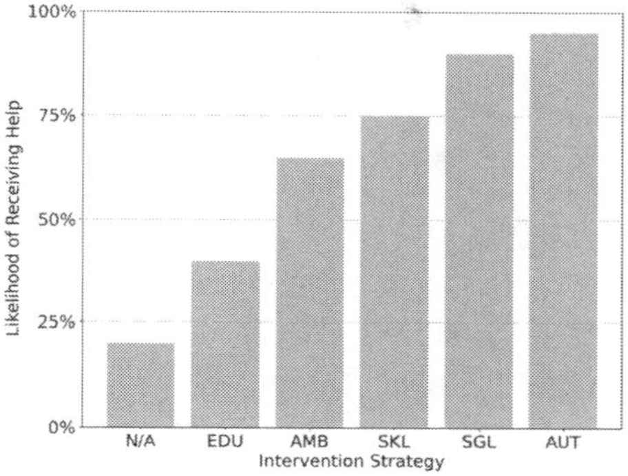

AMB: Reducing Ambiguity (e.g. 'It's an emergency!')

AUT: Authority Figure Takes Charge

EDU: Education on Bystander Effect

N/A: No Intervention (Baseline)

SGL: Singling Out an Individual (e.g. 'You, call 911!')

SKL: Increasing Competence (e.g. First Aid Training)

The chart illustrates that while the probability of receiving help in a situation with multiple bystanders and no clear direction is relatively low (Baseline), targeted interventions can dramatically increase the chances of assistance. The most effective strategies are those that directly counteract the diffusion of responsibility, such as an authority figure taking command or singling out a specific individual to act. These actions create clear personal responsibility and a defined course of action. Strategies that reduce ambiguity (clarifying that it is an emergency) or increase a bystander's perceived competence (e.g., through first-aid training) are also highly effective. Even simply educating people about the bystander effect has a notable positive impact, making them more self-aware and likely to intervene. Please note: These values are principled estimates designed to illustrate the relative effectiveness of different strategies. The actual probability of helping can vary greatly depending on the specific context of the emergency, the number of bystanders, and cultural factors. The chart primarily serves to demonstrate that targeted actions can dramatically overcome the passivity associated with the bystander effect.

4.2.2 Practical Exercises for Strengthening Empathy and Altruism

The ability to feel empathy and compassion is not an immutable trait but a skill that can be deliberately trained. These inner states often drive altruistic actions that stem from a concern for the well-being of others or from moral beliefs [s26]. Strengthening these abilities requires regular and conscious practice, similar to learning an instrument or a sport. One of the most effective methods for this is active perspective-taking. This involves consciously detaching from one's own viewpoint and attempting to understand a situation from the emotional and cognitive perspective of another person.

A specific exercise involves consciously pausing during disagreements or conflict situations. Instead of immediately reacting to the expressed words, focus your attention on uncovering the underlying needs, fears, or hopes of the other person. Ask yourself internally: What is this person feeling right now? What past experiences might shape their reaction? What would I need in their place at this moment? This form of mental training can be applied in various everyday situations. For example, observe a person who appears stressed or upset in public. Instead of judging them, try to find possible reasons for their behavior that have nothing to do with you—perhaps they received bad news or are under immense time pressure. Studies show that consciously inducing compassion through such thought processes significantly increases the willingness to help others [s26]. This exercise not only trains emotional understanding but also reduces hasty judgments and fosters an internal attitude that promotes prosocial behavior.

Beyond these individual cognitive exercises, prosocial behavior can be cultivated through the design of the social environment. People are strongly influenced by the norms and values that are practiced in their surroundings. In families, schools, or workplaces, specific conditions can be created that promote helpfulness and collaboration. This occurs less through appeals and more through lived examples and the establishment of a culture of mutual support [s27]. When children and adolescents observe that helpfulness, cooperation, and fairness are actively practiced in their immediate environment, they internalize these values as a social norm. The same applies to adults in professional or social contexts. Leaders or influential group members who act selflessly and support others set a standard that others follow.

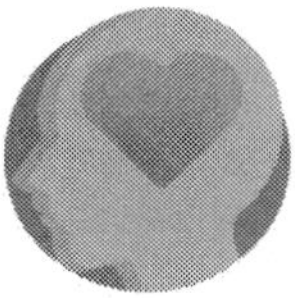

To actively promote such a culture, concrete measures can be taken. These aim to make prosocial behavior visible and an integral part of interactions:
- Initiate conversations about the importance of helpfulness and share personal experiences to destigmatize and make the topic tangible.
- Organize joint charitable activities, such as a fundraising campaign in a club, a neighborhood assistance initiative, or a volunteer project in a company.
- Consciously acknowledge and positively reinforce the prosocial behavior of others to highlight its social value and encourage imitation.

The learning process is deepened through conscious reflection on experienced prosocial actions. After helping or witnessing helpfulness, it is beneficial to take a moment to process the experience. Engaging with questions such as "What impact did my help have on the other person?", "How did my own actions feel?", or "What did I learn about myself and others from the situation?" solidifies the connection between the action and its positive outcome. This reflection strengthens intrinsic motivation and the belief that one can make a difference through their actions, which in turn increases the likelihood of future altruistic engagement [s27]. The combination of cognitive training, the design of a supportive environment, and targeted reflection thus creates a sustainable cycle for promoting empathy and helpfulness.

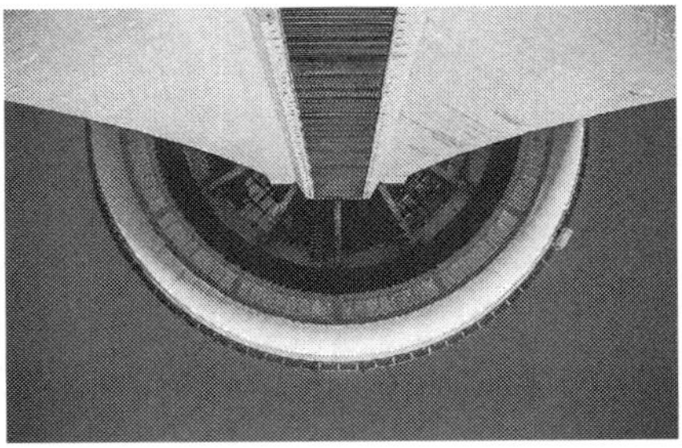

Perspective-taking [i27]

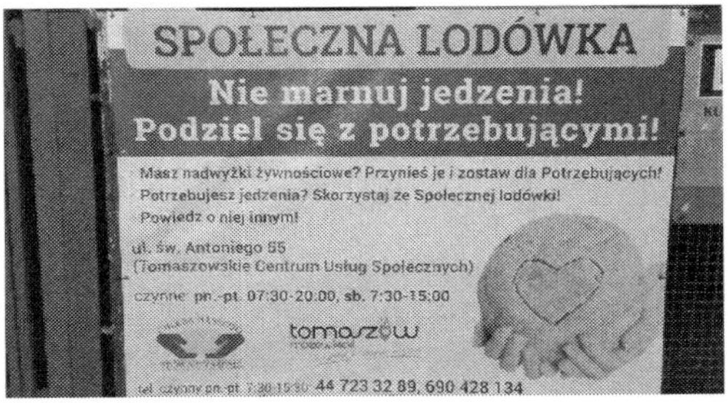

Public-spiritedness [i28]

Good to know

Altruism

Refers to selfless behavior aimed at benefiting others without expecting an immediate or obvious return. It contrasts with actions that are primarily motivated by selfish interests.

Empathy

The ability to not only rationally understand the emotional states of another person (cognitive empathy) but also to vicariously feel with them (emotional empathy). It is considered a fundamental basis for the motivation to help.

Intrinsic Motivation

The inner drive to perform an action because it is perceived as satisfying or meaningful in itself, rather than due to external incentives such as rewards. It is crucial for sustainable engagement.

Perspective-Taking

A cognitive process in which one actively places themselves in the position of another person to understand their thoughts, feelings, and motives. This ability is essential for reducing misunderstandings and responding appropriately to the needs of others.

Social Norm

An unwritten rule of behavior within a group or society that dictates what behavior is considered acceptable or expected. Compliance is often ensured through social pressure or the expectation of approval.

Components of Prosocial Competence

Estimated contribution of different exercise types to the development of overall prosocial competence.

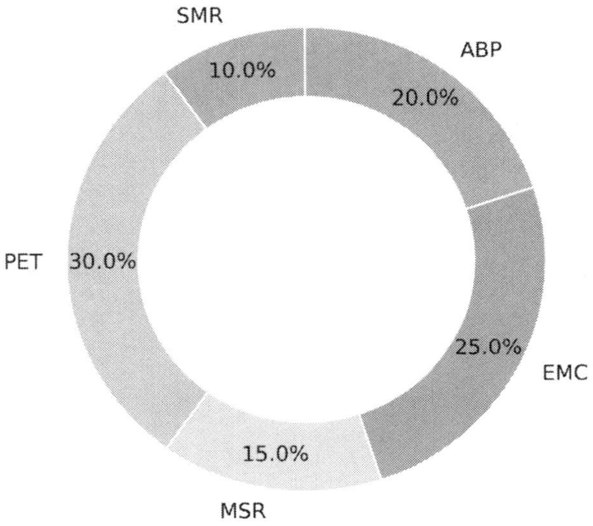

ABP: Altruistic Behavior Practice

EMC: Empathic Concern

MSR: Mindfulness and Self-Regulation

PET: Perspective-Taking

SMR: Social and Moral Reasoning

The chart illustrates that developing prosocial competence is a multifaceted process. The values are conceptual estimates to represent the relative importance of different areas. Cognitive skills, like 'Perspective-Taking' (the ability to understand another's viewpoint), form the largest component. This is closely followed by 'Empathic Concern,' the emotional capacity to feel for others. However, empathy alone is not enough; it must be translated into action, hence the significant contribution of 'Altruistic Behavior Practice.' Supporting these core elements are 'Mindfulness and Self-Regulation,' which are crucial for managing one's own emotional responses to avoid distress or burnout, and 'Social and Moral Reasoning,' which provides the cognitive framework for understanding why helping is important. The key takeaway is that an effective program to enhance prosocial behavior should be holistic, addressing cognitive, emotional, behavioral, and self-regulatory skills in a balanced way.

4.2.3 The Art of Asking for and Accepting Help

Asking for and accepting help are active social skills that represent the counterpart to helpfulness. Although prosocial behavior is highly valued in society, many individuals find it difficult to request or accept support. The reasons for this often lie in deeply rooted psychological mechanisms, such as the protection of one's self-esteem, fear of dependency, or the desire to demonstrate autonomy and competence. However, the inability to seek help can lead to solvable problems escalating and negatively impacting personal well-being. Therefore, learning these skills is beneficial not only for the recipient but also for the social fabric, as it opens up opportunities for potential helpers to act prosocially.

The art of asking begins with overcoming the assumption that others should recognize one's needs and act on their own. This expectation is often unrealistic and leads to disappointment. An effective request for help is instead clear, direct, and specific. Rather than making a vague complaint about having too much work, a precisely formulated request is far more promising. A person asking a colleague for support might say instead of "I'm drowning in work": "Could you please compile the data for the monthly report by 3 PM? That would allow me to finish the presentation on time." Such a request reduces the ambiguity for the potential helper, makes the need concrete, and conveys that the offered help makes a tangible difference. This increases the perceived self-efficacy of the helper and lowers the threshold for agreeing to help.

Another aspect is the psychological framing of the request. Instead of portraying one's need for help as a deficiency, it can be framed as an invitation to collaborate or as an expression of trust. People prefer to help when they feel like competent partners rather than rescuers of a helpless individual. Asking for help signals trust in the other person's abilities and strengthens social bonds. The formulation "I'm stuck on this problem and greatly value your perspective" is more effective than a mere appeal to pity. Successful requests for help often include the following elements:

- **Concreteness**: The problem and the needed support are clearly stated.
- **Directness**: The request is directed specifically to one or more individuals, which reduces diffusion of responsibility.
- **Justification**: A brief explanation of why help is needed and what positive effect it will have increases the helper's motivation.
- **Voluntariness**: The request should be framed in such a way that a "no" is a legitimate response, to avoid pressure and maintain the other person's autonomy.

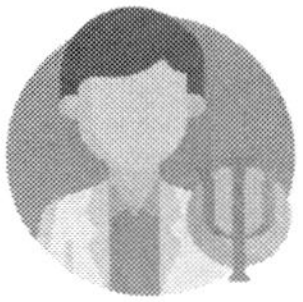

Equally challenging as asking is accepting help, especially when it is offered unsolicited. Accepting support can be perceived as an admission of one's inadequacy or as establishing a social debt. The norm of reciprocity, or the feeling of needing to reciprocate, can lead to the rejection of help out of fear of future obligation. However, rejecting genuinely offered help can be hurtful to the potential helper and dampen their willingness to assist in the future. It devalues their prosocial initiative and can strain the relationship.

Gracefully accepting help is therefore a form of social appreciation. It affirms the helper in their perception and commitment. A simple, sincere expression of thanks is often the most appropriate response. It signals that the gesture is seen and appreciated without implying an immediate reciprocation. Accepting help is thus not a passive act but an active affirmation of social connection. It allows the helper to experience the positive emotions associated with altruistic actions, such as enhanced self-esteem and a sense of purpose. By learning to accept help, one actively contributes to fostering a culture of reciprocity, where giving and receiving are understood as equally important components of a functioning social exchange. Ultimately, this closes the circle of prosocial behavior: the competence to ask for help and to accept it is the necessary prerequisite for helpfulness to be effective.

Good to know

Ambiguity

Describes the uncertainty or vagueness of a situation. In emergencies, ambiguity leads potential helpers to be unsure whether an emergency exists or what type of support is needed, which can result in hesitant behavior or inaction.

Diffusion of Responsibility

Describes the psychological phenomenon that the subjectively felt responsibility of an individual to help decreases as more people are present. Each individual assumes that another will intervene, which reduces the likelihood of actual assistance.

Norm of Reciprocity

Refers to a universal social rule that states one should reciprocate for received goods or favors. This norm stabilizes social relationships but can also complicate the acceptance of help if the receiving person fears they cannot repay the debt.

Self-Efficacy

Refers to a person's belief in their ability to successfully manage a specific task or challenge. In the context of helping, it is the helper's belief that their intervention can indeed make a positive and effective contribution.

The Art of Asking for Help

Likelihood of receiving help, based on social closeness and the clarity of the request.

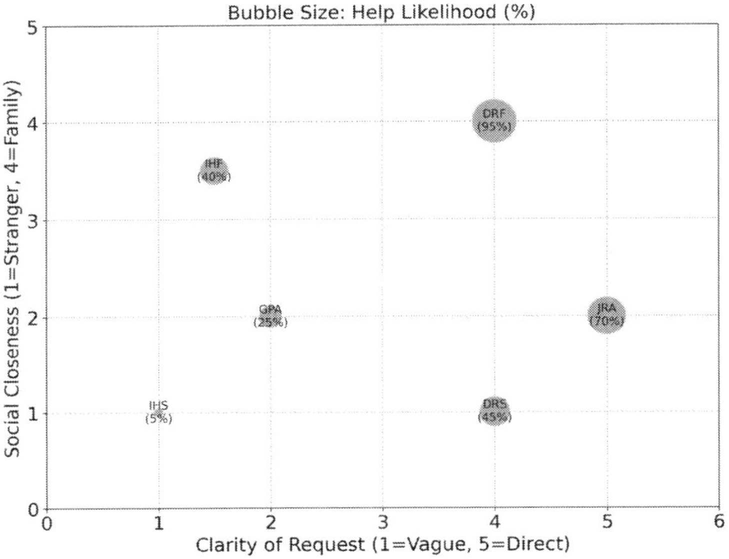

Blasengröße: Help Likelihood (%)

DRF: Direct Request to Family

DRS: Direct Request to Stranger

GPA: General Plea to Acquaintance

IHF: Indirect Hint to Friend

IHS: Indirect Hint to Stranger

JRA: Justified Request to Acquaintance

These data are estimations designed to illustrate fundamental principles of social psychology. The chart shows a clear trend: the likelihood of receiving help (bubble size) increases with both the social closeness to the person being asked (Y-axis) and the clarity and directness of the request (X-axis). A vague, indirect hint to a stranger has a very low probability of success, as the request may not even be recognized as such. In contrast, a direct, personal request to a close friend is almost always successful. Interestingly, even with strangers, a clear and direct request significantly increases the chances of receiving help compared to an indirect one. The key takeaway is that for help to be given, it must first be clearly requested. While close relationships provide a buffer for less clear communication, directness is a universally effective strategy for activating prosocial behavior.

4. 3 Dealing with Aggression and Partnership Conflicts

Aggression and recurring conflicts pose a serious threat to the stability and intimacy of partnerships. They often arise from a combination of learned behavioral patterns, personal traits such as low impulse control, and the pursuit of control, leading to destructive cycles. This chapter analyzes these dynamics and provides the psychological tools for constructive engagement. It highlights the causes of aggressive behavior and presents concrete tools for emotional regulation and de-escalating communication, which facilitate joint problem-solving. Understanding these mechanisms and techniques empowers individuals to break destructive patterns and actively transform conflicts into opportunities for greater connection.

> *The solution for partner aggression does not lie in controlling the partner, but in mastering one's own learned reactions.*

> *Conquer anger with love, evil with good, meanness with generosity, and lies with truth.*

Gautama Buddha

Dhammapada
Ch. 17, Verse 223

This teaching from the Dhammapada offers a psychologically sophisticated strategy for conflict resolution. Instead of responding to aggression with more aggression (a common escalatory cycle), it advocates for a counter-intuitive approach: meeting negative actions with their prosocial opposites. This principle resonates with cognitive-behavioral techniques that focus on breaking negative interaction patterns by consciously choosing a different, more constructive response, thereby de-escalating conflict and fostering reconciliation.

4.3.1 Analysis of Triggers for Aggressive Behavior

Aggressive behavior in partnerships often stems from the desire to exert power and control over the partner. It rarely manifests as isolated, uncontrolled outbursts, but rather as a behavioral pattern aimed at enforcing one's will and dominating the other [s28]. Therefore, the analysis of triggers begins with examining the underlying motivation behind the behavior.

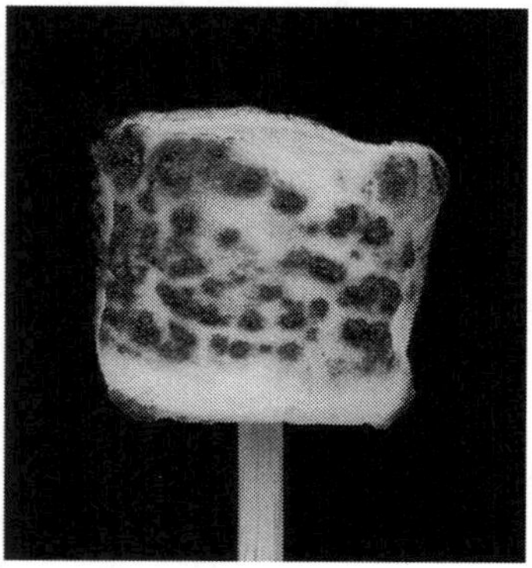

Impulse control [i29]

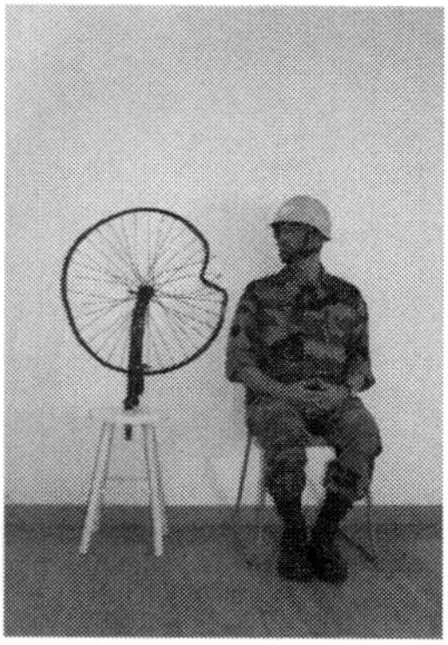

Cycle of violence [i30]

Social psychology provides explanatory models, such as the social learning theory. This theory posits that aggressive behavior is not innate but learned. Individuals adopt behaviors they observe in their environment, particularly when these behaviors lead to success or are rewarded. The intergenerational transmission of violence serves as evidence for this mechanism. Children who witness conflicts resolved through verbal or physical aggression in their homes internalize this pattern as a legitimate or even normal strategy for problem-solving. They learn through observation that aggression is a means to satisfy needs or to end a confrontation, increasing the likelihood that they will reproduce this behavior in their own later relationships, whether as perpetrators or victims [s28].

In addition to these learned patterns, individual personality traits also contribute to the emergence of aggression. Certain traits can lower the threshold for aggressive actions. These include:

- A pronounced jealousy that misinterprets harmless interactions of the partner as threats to the relationship.
- Low impulse control, making it difficult to respond calmly to frustration or provocation.
- The tendency to consistently blame others for one's own mistakes or conflicts and to see oneself as a victim of circumstances [s28].

These personality factors create a fertile ground for conflicts to escalate more easily. A person who is quickly jealous and simultaneously struggles to control their impulses may respond to a perceived threat not with a clarifying conversation but with anger and accusations. If this person also tends to place all the blame on the partner, de-escalation becomes nearly impossible, as their own role in the conflict is not reflected upon.

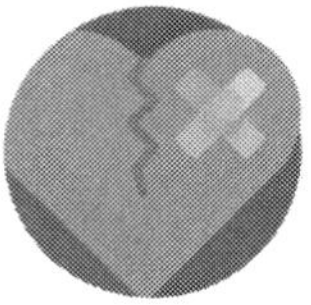

This interplay of the desire for control, learned behavioral patterns, and personal risk factors often culminates in a recurring cycle of violence. This cycle typically consists of several phases that repeat and dynamically shape the relationship. Initially, tension builds, characterized by minor conflicts, irritability, and subtle displays of power. This phase culminates in an acute aggressive episode marked by verbal or physical attacks. Often, this is followed by a phase of remorse and reconciliation, during which the aggressive person expresses regret, makes promises, and behaves overly affectionately. Finally, a calm phase ensues, during which conflicts seem to be resolved, before the cycle begins anew with a fresh buildup of tension [s28].

For the person acting aggressively, analyzing these phases serves as a tool for self-reflection. When does the tension begin? What thoughts and feelings precede the escalation? The conscious awareness of these recurring patterns in one's behavior allows for early intervention before the situation spirals out of control. For instance, recognizing the first signs of internal tension—a quickened pulse, tense muscles, circling negative thoughts—can serve as a signal to consciously leave the situation, take a break, and only resume the conversation once one's emotional arousal has subsided.

Good to know

Cycle of Violence

A model that describes the recurring phases in violent relationships. The regular sequence of tension buildup, outbreak of violence, and subsequent remorse or reconciliation phase explains why it is often difficult for those affected to end the relationship, as the positive phases repeatedly evoke hope for improvement.

Intergenerational Transmission

Refers to the often unconscious transfer of behaviors, emotional patterns, and relationship conflicts from one generation to the next within a family. Thus, experienced conflict styles of parents can shape how one later conducts their own partnership disputes.

Social Learning Theory

A theory that explains that behavior is learned not only through personal experiences but also through the observation of others and the consequences of their actions. In the context of conflicts, this means that aggressive resolution strategies can be adopted if perceived as successful in others.

Frequency of Aggression Triggers in Partnerships

Estimated frequency of common conflict triggers that can lead to aggressive behavior.

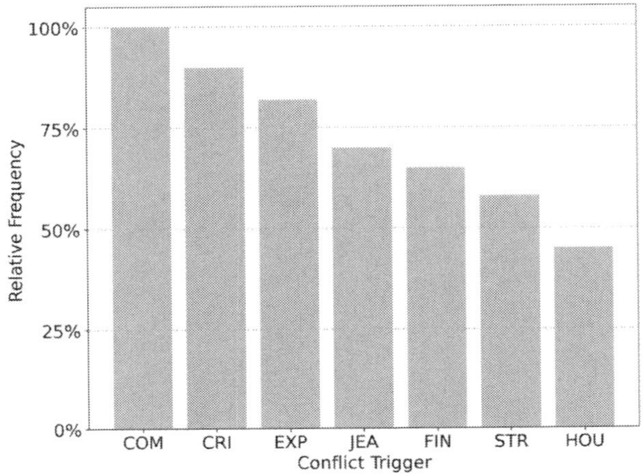

COM: Communication Issues

CRI: Perceived Criticism

EXP: Unfulfilled Expectations

FIN: Financial Stress

HOU: Household Disagreements

JEA: Jealousy

STR: External Stress (Work/Family)

This chart illustrates the estimated frequency of various triggers for aggressive behavior within partnerships. The data clearly indicates that communication-related issues, such as misunderstandings and poor expression, are the most significant catalysts for conflict. Closely following are feelings of being criticized and having unfulfilled expectations, both of which are often consequences of ineffective communication. Emotional factors like jealousy and external pressures such as financial or work-related stress also emerge as major contributors. Even daily practicalities like disagreements over household chores represent a notable source of tension. In conclusion, these estimations highlight that aggressive conflicts are rarely caused by a single factor, but rather a combination of poor communication patterns, emotional vulnerabilities, and external stressors. It is important to note that these figures are illustrative estimates intended to show general principles from social psychological findings; actual frequencies can vary significantly between individual relationships.

4.3.2 Methods for Emotion Regulation and Impulse Control

The ability to manage one's own emotions and control impulses is a learnable skill that counteracts destructive behavior patterns in conflict situations. Instead of suppressing emotions, which often leads to an uncontrolled outburst later, effective methods aim to change or consciously channel the emotional response itself. A central technique for this is cognitive reappraisal. This involves mentally reinterpreting a potentially conflict-triggering situation to diminish its emotional impact. Instead of immediately interpreting a partner's lateness as a sign of disrespect—an interpretation that generates immediate anger—the situation can be reframed. Possible alternative explanations, such as unforeseen traffic delays or an urgent work call, transform the feeling of anger into concern or patience. This mental step creates a distance between the triggering event and the emotional reaction, opening up options for action beyond aggressive impulses.

A prerequisite for such reappraisal processes is the ability to accurately recognize and name one's own feelings. Research shows that particularly men, who find it difficult to clearly identify their emotions, exhibit a higher risk of violent behavior in relationships [s29]. A diffuse, unpleasant arousal that cannot be differentiated into specific feelings such as disappointment, fear, or offense is more likely to discharge in an impulsive, aggressive act. Difficulties in emotion regulation are directly related to the use of violence, as uncontrolled feelings are often experienced as unbearable and seem to be ended by an aggressive act [s29]. It is helpful to consciously pause and self-question: "What exactly am I feeling at this moment? Is it anger, or is it the fear of not being heard? Is it annoyance, or is it disappointment over an unmet need?" This emotional clarity is the first step in understanding the actual source of the conflict and responding appropriately, rather than blindly attacking.

In addition to these cognitive approaches, there are behavior-based techniques that directly aim to reduce physical arousal. These are useful when the emotional intensity is so high that cognitive reappraisal is no longer possible.

- An agreed-upon "time-out" is not a punishment or a conversation interruption, but a conscious break to allow the physiological stress response to subside. Rational thinking is severely restricted during high emotional arousal due to the activation of older brain regions (such as the amygdala). A break of 20 to 30 minutes gives the body time to reduce stress hormones and return control to the prefrontal cortex—the seat of reason and impulse control.

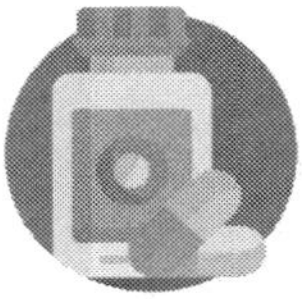

- During this time-out, it is effective to focus on one's own body rather than dwelling on the conflict mentally. Techniques such as diaphragmatic breathing, which involves deep abdominal breathing, or the targeted tensing and relaxing of muscle groups (progressive muscle relaxation), have been shown to lower heart rate and blood pressure.
- Even a brief but intense physical activity, such as climbing stairs or doing push-ups, can help release pent-up aggressive energy in a non-harmful way and clear the mind.

The combination of these methods—cognitive reappraisal, emotional differentiation, and behavior-based de-escalation—enables a constructive approach to conflict situations. Instead of reacting impulsively to a stimulus and undermining long-term relationship goals such as trust and intimacy, a space for conscious action is created. Research confirms that targeted interventions to improve these regulatory skills can reduce the frequency of partner violence, as they directly address the mechanisms that favor impulsive reactions [s29]. Learning these techniques empowers a person to actively shape their reactions rather than being controlled by them.

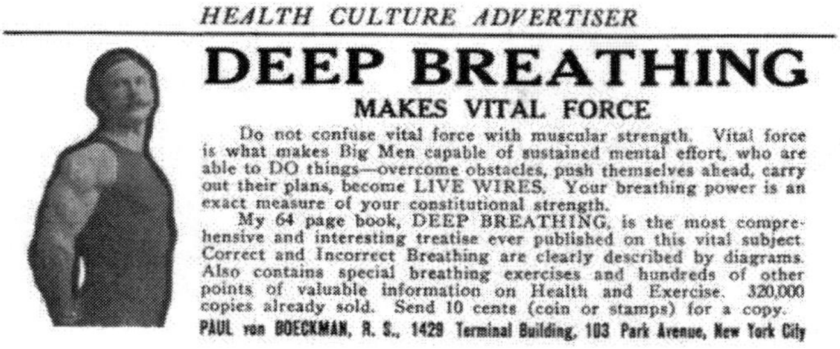

Diaphragmatic breathing [i31]

Good to know

Cognitive Reappraisal

A mental technique in which the meaning of a situation is consciously altered to control the associated emotional response. This process helps to break negative thought spirals before they lead to strong feelings such as anger or frustration. It is a core component of therapies aimed at changing harmful behavior patterns.

Prefrontal Cortex

The front part of the cerebral cortex responsible for higher mental functions. These include planning actions, weighing consequences, and consciously controlling impulses. A well-functioning control by this area is crucial for acting thoughtfully rather than reactively in emotional moments.

Progressive Muscle Relaxation

A procedure in which individual muscle groups are deliberately tensed and then relaxed. This method trains body awareness and the ability to distinguish between tension and relaxation. As a result, the physical signs of emerging stress can be recognized early and alleviated through conscious relaxation.

Effectiveness of Impulse Control Methods

Comparison of the long-term effectiveness of various emotion regulation techniques.

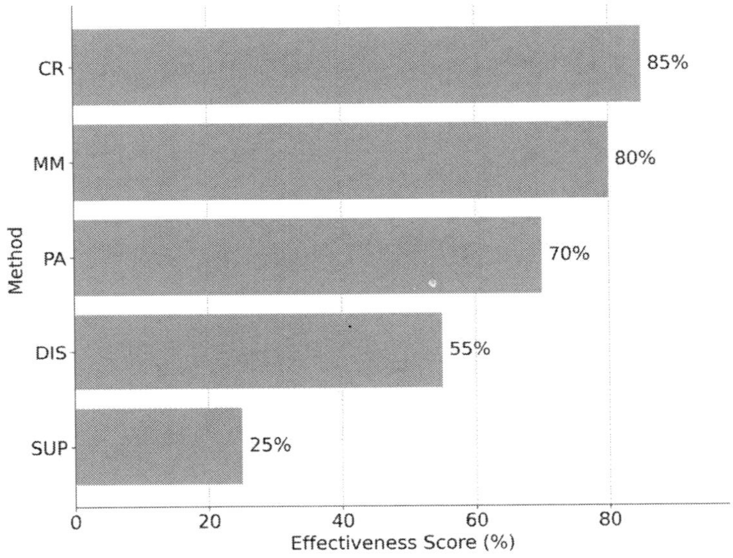

CR: Cognitive Reappraisal

MM: Mindfulness and Meditation

SUP: Expressive Suppression

DIS: Distraction

PA: Physical Activity

The chart illustrates the varying long-term effectiveness of different strategies for managing aggressive impulses. Cognitive-based methods, such as Cognitive Reappraisal and Mindfulness, demonstrate the highest efficacy, suggesting they facilitate fundamental and lasting changes in emotional response. Physical Activity is also a very potent tool, particularly for immediate de-escalation. Distraction offers a temporary, moderately effective solution. In stark contrast, Expressive Suppression is shown to be the least effective approach, highlighting that simply inhibiting emotional expression is not a viable long-term strategy for conflict resolution. It is important to note that these values are estimates designed to represent general findings in psychological research and to illustrate the principles of effectiveness, rather than being precise data from a single comparative study.

4.3.3 Application of Negotiation Strategies in Couple Relationships

Conflicts in couple relationships can be understood as negotiation processes in which two parties attempt to reconcile their differing interests and needs. The success of these negotiations depends less on who is "right" and more on the communication strategies employed. A common cause of the escalation of disputes is the resort to accusatory communication patterns. The use of phrases that attribute sole responsibility or blame for a problem to the other party is demonstrably associated with relational aggression and a decline in relationship quality [s30]. Such "you-messages" trigger an immediate defensive reaction in the partner, as they are perceived as personal attacks rather than invitations to collaboratively solve a problem. The conversation shifts from the issue at hand to a personal confrontation, where both sides attempt to defend themselves or retaliate.

Constructive negotiation begins with a conscious change in these language patterns. The focus shifts from accusing the partner to describing one's own perceptions, feelings, and needs. A statement like "You never take care of the household" provokes resistance. An alternative formulation shifts the emphasis: "I feel overwhelmed with the housework and worry that I have to manage everything alone. I wish we could find a solution for a fairer division of tasks." This approach can be compared to moving from an indictment to a joint project plan. It removes the personal sharpness from the dispute and opens a space for cooperative solutions, as it centers on the shared problem rather than the partner's character. This change in communication does not undermine the partner's autonomy, but strengthens the connection by demonstrating that a common goal is being pursued [s30].

Beyond avoiding destructive patterns, actively introducing positive engagement is a factor for successful conflict resolution. Positive engagement includes behaviors that signal to the partner that their perspective is heard and valued, even when there is disagreement on the issue. This encompasses active listening without interruptions, showing empathy for the other's feelings, and validating their viewpoint ("I can understand why you see it that way."). Studies show that a high level of positive engagement during a dispute increases the relationship satisfaction of both partners [s31]. It creates a climate of safety in which both sides are willing to open up and show vulnerability, which is a prerequisite for identifying the actual, deeper needs.

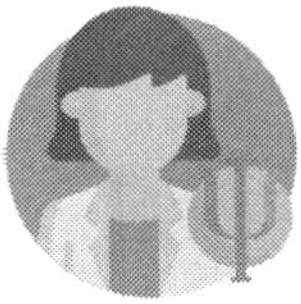

The dynamics of these interactions are complex. Research indicates that particularly the positive engagement of the woman can have a strong positive influence on the satisfaction of both partners. Conversely, psychological aggression—such as derogatory remarks, sarcasm, or demonstrative silence—can be toxic and lead to a significant deterioration of the conversational climate. This is particularly detrimental when expressed in discussions about the man's concerns or problems [s31]. A productive negotiation therefore does not focus on rigid positions ("I want you to do this"), but rather on the underlying interests ("I want to feel understood and supported"). The goal is not to win over the partner, but to find a solution that considers the needs of both sides and strengthens the relationship as a whole. The application of these negotiation strategies transforms a conflict from a fight against each other into a joint effort to strengthen the bond and create a stable foundation for future differences.

Good to know

Escalation

Describes the process by which a conflict increases in intensity and hostility. Often, a negative spiral develops, where one negative remark is met with an even more negative response. The original issue is abandoned, and the argument expands to other, often past topics.

Positive Engagement

A communication style that actively aims to create a supportive and appreciative atmosphere. Research shows that a ratio of at least five positive to one negative interaction during a conflict is a strong indicator of a stable and happy partnership.

Psychological Aggression

Includes verbal and nonverbal actions aimed at emotionally hurting, humiliating, or controlling another person. In contrast to an open confrontation over a factual issue, it attacks the psyche and self-esteem of the partner.

Relational Aggression

A form of harmful behavior aimed at damaging a person's social relationships or sense of belonging. This often occurs through indirect means such as targeted ignoring, social exclusion, or spreading rumors to undermine the partner's social standing.

Negotiation Strategy and Relationship Satisfaction

This chart shows the correlation between the quality of conflict negotiation strategies and the level of relationship satisfaction.

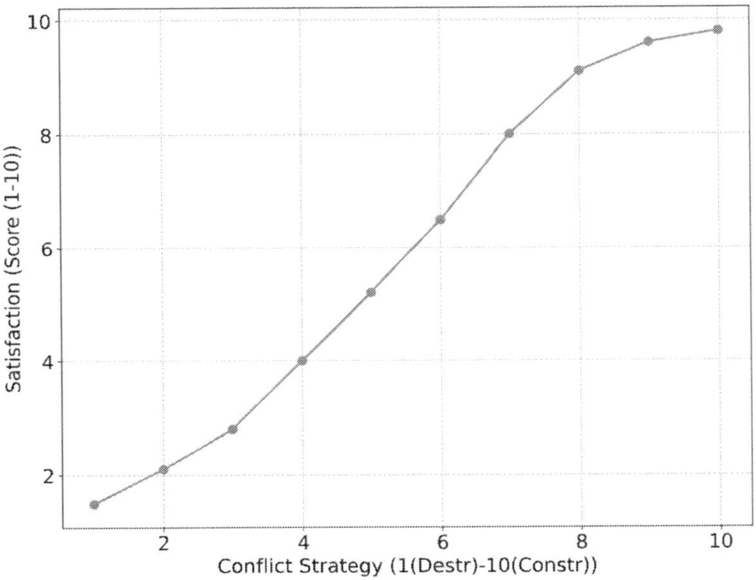

The diagram illustrates a strong positive correlation between the type of negotiation strategy used in conflicts and the overall satisfaction within the partnership. At the lower end of the x-axis, where strategies are destructive or aggressive, relationship satisfaction is consistently very low. As strategies become more neutral or avoidant, satisfaction increases moderately, suggesting that avoiding conflict is preferable to destructive engagement, but not a path to high satisfaction. The most significant jump in satisfaction occurs when couples move towards collaborative and constructive strategies. This indicates that active listening, validation, and a focus on finding mutually beneficial solutions are key drivers of a highly satisfying and stable partnership. It's important to note that these values are principled estimations intended to illustrate this well-documented psychological dynamic, not data from a specific, single study.

Review - 4. Interpersonal Relationships: Attraction, Conflicts, and Prosocial Behavior

The social psychological examination of interpersonal relationships reveals a fascinating yet often unconscious choreography of our social lives. From initial attraction to conflict resolution, we rarely operate on a purely rational stage. Instead, we are guided by subtle forces such as spatial proximity, perceived similarity, and unconscious judgments about a person's appearance. The true art lies in understanding these hidden mechanisms and viewing them not as immutable fate but as malleable material. Rather than passively allowing yourself to be socialized by the architecture of an office or the random seating arrangement in a seminar room, you can proactively seek social spaces that align with your values and interests. Join a club, attend courses, or engage in volunteer work in areas that matter to you. This ensures that the effect of mere presence operates among individuals with whom a deeper similarity on crucial life issues is likely. At the same time, this requires vigilance to unmask the attractiveness halo effect within yourself. Ask yourself pointedly: Is my positive assessment of this person based on their specific behavior and contributions, or am I being blinded by a likable appearance? This conscious self-reflection is the first step toward becoming an active shaper of your relationships rather than a passive object of social forces.

This active role is particularly challenged in critical moments, whether in a public emergency or a private conflict. The bystander effect teaches us that passivity is contagious. Overcoming this paralysis begins with a conscious mental act: the decision that the responsibility lies right here and now with you. Instead of hoping that someone else will intervene, you can reverse the dynamics by breaking the anonymity of the crowd. A direct, clear address—"You in the red jacket, please call the ambulance!"—transforms passive observers into active helpers and creates a temporary, capable community. This ability to take responsibility is also key to asking for help. Many hesitate, fearing they will appear weak or needy. Yet a precise and well-founded request is not a sign of weakness but of competence and trust. You honor the other person by believing they can be a valuable support. Accepting help, in turn, is an equally important social skill that affirms the helper's effectiveness and strengthens the social bond, rather than weakening it through false shame or pride.

In our closest relationships, where conflicts are inevitable, the ability to self-regulate proves crucial. Instead of reacting to provocation with a reflexive counterattack that inevitably leads to a destructive spiral, it is essential to create an inner space between stimulus and response. The most important practice for this is the agreed-upon "time-out." It is not a conversation interruption but a strategic pause to allow the physiological stress response to subside and to return rational thinking to the forefront. In this pause, you can cognitively reassess the situation: instead of interpreting your partner's action as a personal attack, look for alternative, more benevolent explanations. Once the emotional wave has receded, you can resume the conversation with a cooperative problem-solving attitude. Shifting from accusatory "you-messages" to descriptive "I-messages" that articulate one's own feelings and needs transforms the conflict from a struggle against each other into a joint search for a solution that considers both partners' needs and strengthens the relationship.

Ultimately, the cultivation of successful interpersonal relationships is a learnable skill based on awareness and conscious action. The insights of social psychology provide us with a map of the invisible forces that shape our interactions. By learning to read this map, we can stop drifting aimlessly through our social world. We gain the ability to chart our own course, actively forge connections, demonstrate responsibility in critical moments, and view conflicts as opportunities for growth. This is not a one-time act but a continuous process of self-reflection and practice, leading to an invaluable gain: authentic, stable, and fulfilling relationships.

5. Applied Social Psychology: Consumer and Behavior Control in Everyday Life

Why do we automatically reach for certain products in the supermarket, even though they weren't on our shopping list? Social psychology not only provides theoretical explanations for human behavior but also finds practical application in our daily lives. From the strategic placement of goods to the design of social campaigns, companies and organizations utilize psychological insights to influence our behavior. At the same time, these methods open pathways to address societal challenges such as discrimination and bias. This chapter demonstrates how social psychological principles act as powerful tools for behavior control—often without our awareness.

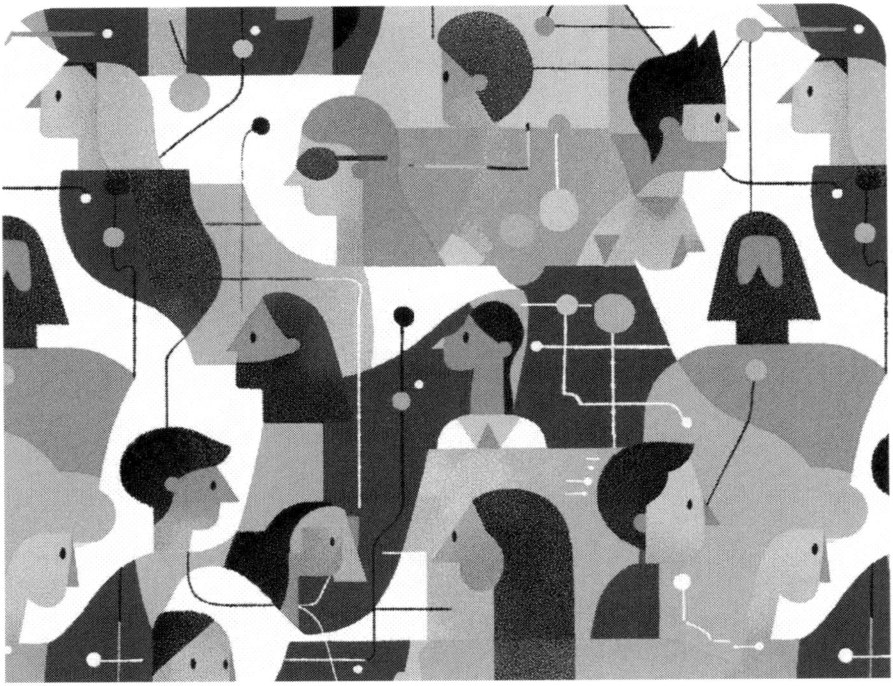

The Psychology of Persuasion

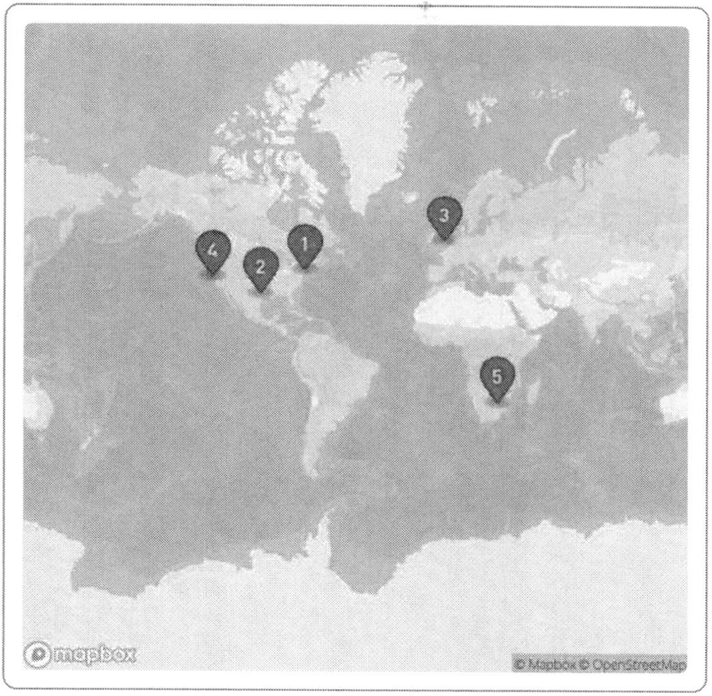

A map of influential campaigns and initiatives that successfully used social psychological principles to shape behavior.

1 **Doyle Dane Bernbach (DDB), New York, NY**
Birthplace of Volkswagen's 'Think Small' campaign (1959). This campaign revolutionized advertising by using honesty and the inoculation effect. Instead of hiding the car's small size, DDB embraced it as a virtue, preemptively addressing consumer doubts to build trust and credibility in an era of large American cars.

2 **Texas Department of Transportation, Austin, TX**
Origin of the 'Don't Mess with Texas' anti-littering campaign (1986). The campaign successfully used social identity theory by linking anti-littering behavior to a tough, proud Texan identity. Featuring Texas celebrities, it made not littering a powerful in-group norm, transforming it from a civic duty into an act of state pride.

3 **Sport England, London, UK**
Headquarters for the 'This Girl Can' campaign (2015), a public health initiative to encourage women in sports. The campaign powerfully used social proof by featuring real, relatable women of all body types celebrating their activity. This normalized exercise and directly addressed the 'fear of judgment,' a major barrier for many women.

4 **Goodby Silverstein & Partners, San Francisco, CA**
The ad agency that created the iconic 'Got Milk?' campaign (1993). The campaign masterfully employed the principle of scarcity or deprivation. Instead of showing the joys of drinking milk, it focused on the frustrating moment when you desperately need it but don't have it, making its absence acutely felt and motivating purchase.

5 **De Beers Group, Johannesburg, South Africa**
A key hub for De Beers, the company behind the 'A Diamond is Forever' campaign (1947). This campaign manufactured a social norm by linking diamonds to eternal love, making the diamond ring an essential symbol of engagement. It established a powerful tradition based on the principles of commitment and social proof.

5. 1 Consumer Psychology: Understanding and Controlling Purchasing Decisions

Purchase decisions are subject to a variety of psychological influences that often go unnoticed. Advertising messages evoke needs, brand loyalty fosters trust, and the design of the shopping environment directs attention. Emotional states and impulsive reactions interact with external stimuli, systematically shaping consumer behavior. This chapter reveals the mechanisms behind these processes. It analyzes how cognitive biases, heuristics, and the architecture of decision-making situations guide our choices without formally restricting freedom. Understanding these effects is key to comprehending purchase decisions and enhancing one's autonomy as a consumer.

A purchasing decision is rarely the result of free, rational consideration, but rather the predictable reaction to a deliberately designed environment that activates our unconscious thought patterns and emotional needs.

> *Often when looking at a mass of things for sale, he would say to himself, "How many things I have no need of!"*

Socrates

Diogenes Laertius

Socrates' reflection provides a timeless counterpoint to the mechanisms of consumer psychology. While marketing and advertising focus on creating desire and a sense of need, Socrates champions self-awareness and rational assessment. His habit of questioning his own material wants is a form of cognitive defense against persuasive appeals, representing the critical consumer who consciously evaluates true needs versus manufactured desires—a central tension in the study of consumption.

5.1.1 The Effect of Advertising Messages and Brand Loyalty

Advertising messages aim to evoke or enhance a desire for products or services in the minds of consumers. They utilize psychological mechanisms to actively motivate purchasing decisions [s32]. This influence occurs not only through traditional media such as television or print advertisements but increasingly also directly at the point of sale or in digital environments. The design of the immediate sales environment, including visual stimuli such as packaging design or product placement, interacts with advertising messages and can increase the willingness to buy. The perception of sales promotions, such as discounts or special offers, has a direct impact on purchasing behavior, as they trigger expectations and feelings of urgency among consumers [s32].

Psychological factors are highly relevant in the purchasing decision process, as they shape consumer intentions. Emotional states such as joy, stress, or the need for reward can increase receptiveness to advertising messages and lead to unreflective purchases. This effect is particularly evident in impulsive buying behavior. Here, the purchasing decision is made spontaneously and often unplanned at the point of sale, triggered by a combination of the consumer's internal state and external incentives. An attractively presented candy at the checkout after a tiring workday can trigger such an impulse, as the advertising message of quick reward meets a receptive emotional state.

Beyond the short-term activation of purchasing impulses, market communication pursues a more sustainable goal: the establishment of brand loyalty. This occurs when consumers repeatedly have positive experiences with a brand and develop an emotional connection to it. Brand loyalty is more than just the habit of purchasing a specific product; it is a deeper, emotionally anchored preference based on trust, identification, and positive associations. This emotional charge of a brand leads consumers to build a relationship with it that goes beyond mere utility. To become more aware of this subtle influence, self-reflection can be helpful: Which brands do I purchase regularly and why? Often, the reasons lie not solely in product quality but in the positive feelings or sense of belonging that the brand conveys.

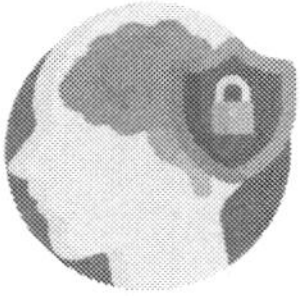

Once established, brand loyalty acts as a cognitive filter. Advertising messages from the preferred brand are received more positively and with less critical distance, while advertisements for competing products lose effectiveness or are completely ignored. Brand-loyal consumers develop an emotional connection through repeated positive experiences, which sustainably shapes their perception and behavior [s32]. For them, the brand fulfills multiple functions simultaneously:
- It reduces the cognitive load in the purchasing decision, as not all alternatives need to be re-evaluated with each purchase.
- It creates trust and lowers the perceived purchase risk, as the quality and expected experience are known.
- It generates a sense of security through consistency and can support the consumer's self-image through identification with the brand values.

Thus, advertising messages and brand loyalty are in a reciprocal relationship. While advertising establishes the initial contact and sets short-term purchasing incentives, brand loyalty solidifies the customer relationship in the long term. It makes consumers more loyal and simultaneously more receptive to future messages from the familiar brand, closing the cycle of perception, purchase, and confirmation.

Good to know

Cognitive Filter

A mental mechanism that selectively controls the perception of information. Existing attitudes and beliefs, such as brand loyalty, determine which messages are attended to and deemed relevant, while others are ignored. This serves to protect against information overload.

Impulsive Buying Behavior

A purchase made without prior planning and often in response to an immediate stimulus. This behavior arises from an internal conflict between the desire for immediate reward and long-term self-control. Mental exhaustion can weaken the ability to self-regulate and favor such behavior.

Market Communication

The totality of all measures a company uses to engage with its target audiences. The goal is to establish a consistent and positive image of a brand or product in people's minds, thereby influencing their attitudes and behaviors.

Sales Promotion

Time-limited incentives aimed at triggering an immediate purchase response. They utilize psychological effects such as the scarcity principle, where limited availability increases the perceived value of an offer and accelerates decision-making.

Impact of Advertising Channels on Brand Loyalty

Effectiveness of various channels in fostering long-term customer brand loyalty.

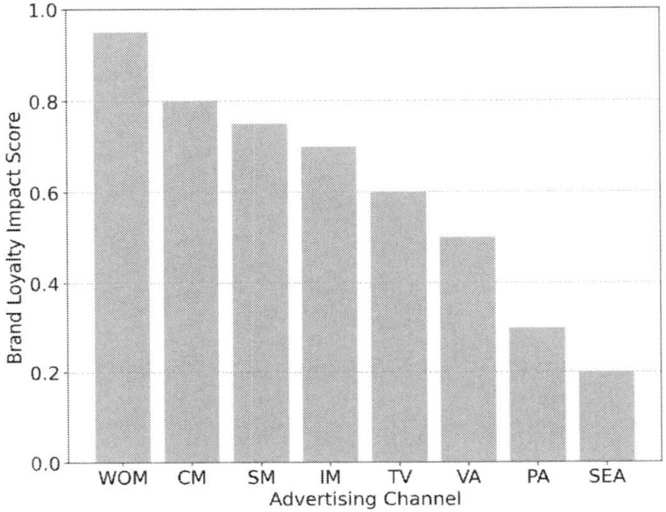

CM: Content Marketing
PA: Print Ads
SM: Social Media
VA: Online Video Ads
IM: Influencer Marketing
SEA: Search Ads (SEA)
TV: TV Advertising
WOM: Word-of-Mouth

The chart illustrates that advertising channels fostering personal connection, trust, and community are most effective at building deep brand loyalty. Word-of-Mouth, based on personal trust, is shown to be the most powerful driver. Content and Social Media marketing follow, as they allow brands to build a relationship over time by providing value and fostering a community. In contrast, channels with one-way communication or a purely transactional focus show a lower impact. While TV ads can create emotional connections through storytelling, they are less interactive. Search Ads are highly effective for immediate sales conversions but contribute little to a lasting emotional bond. These figures are estimates based on general principles of consumer psychology. They are intended to illustrate the fundamental mechanisms of how different advertising channels affect brand loyalty, rather than representing precise empirical data from a specific study.

5.1.2 Use of heuristics and cognitive biases in shopping

To cope with the flood of information in purchasing decisions, the human brain relies on mental shortcuts known as heuristics. These judgment heuristics reduce cognitive effort by breaking down complex problems into simple rules of thumb. Although these processes are efficient, they systematically lead to cognitive biases that subtly influence purchasing behavior and are strategically exploited by marketing strategies. Understanding these mechanisms allows consumers to make their purchasing decisions more consciously and to recognize manipulations.

A common cognitive bias is the anchoring heuristic. Here, the first piece of information a consumer receives serves as a mental "anchor" that influences all subsequent evaluations. In retail, this is often exploited by presenting a high, crossed-out "original price" next to a lower sale price. The high price anchors the perception of the product's value, making the reduced price appear particularly advantageous, even if the absolute value of the item is lower. To counteract this effect, it is helpful to research the actual market value of comparable items *before* evaluating the discounted offer. This sets a personal, more realistic anchor point that clarifies the proportionality of the offer.

The availability heuristic leads to information that is easily retrievable from memory being rated as more relevant or likely. Frequent advertising presence of a product in various media ensures that the brand is more mentally present at the crucial moment of purchase. A consumer who has repeatedly encountered the message that a particular detergent delivers "brilliant white laundry" is more likely to remember this product in the supermarket aisle and rate its advertised property as accurate, without having made objective comparisons. The sheer repetition of the message increases its perceived credibility and availability.

Closely related is the scarcity principle, which states that products are perceived as more valuable when their availability is limited. Phrases like "For a limited time only" or "While supplies last" create urgency and the fear of missing out on a special opportunity (Fear of Missing Out, FOMO). This artificial scarcity shifts the focus from the actual product benefit to the impending unavailability and can lead to hasty purchasing decisions.

Furthermore, the framing effect influences decision-making by presenting the same fact in a different light through different wording. The label "80% lean meat" on a package appears more positive and healthier than the factually identical label "20% fat content." Although the information is the same, the positive framing elicits a more favorable evaluation and increases the likelihood of purchase. Similarly, the representativeness heuristic operates: consumers infer overall quality from superficial characteristics. An elaborate, elegantly designed package suggests a high-quality product, even if the contents are identical to a cheaper competitor's product. The packaging is seen as representative of the quality.

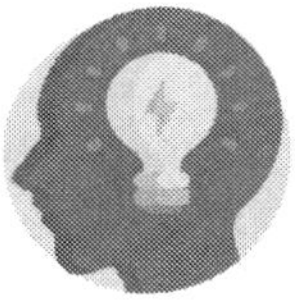

Another mechanism is the endowment effect. People tend to value an item more highly once they own it—or even just feel they own it. Free trial periods, test drives, or the simple prompt in a store to hold a product create a psychological attachment. The subsequent return or non-purchase is then felt as a loss, influencing the purchasing decision in favor of the product. These mental shortcuts and perception distortions are not errors in thinking but expressions of the brain's efficiency. However, knowledge of their existence and functioning enables consumers to recognize the underlying automatism and to make their decisions more rationally and autonomously.

Good to know

Availability Heuristic

A mental shortcut in which the probability or importance of an event is judged based on how easily examples can be retrieved from memory. Particularly emotional or recently experienced events are mentally more accessible, distorting judgment.

Cognitive Bias

A systematic pattern of deviation from rational judgment. Such thought patterns are not individual errors but predictable tendencies that occur in all people, influencing not only purchasing decisions but also social perceptions and memories.

Fear of Missing Out

The widespread concern of missing out on a rewarding or important social experience that others are currently having. This feeling is amplified by social media and can lead to impulsive consumption to gain a sense of belonging.

Representativeness Heuristic

The tendency to evaluate the probability of events based on how much they resemble a prototype or stereotype. Important statistical base information is often neglected, leading to misjudgments of actual quality or characteristics.

Impact of Heuristics on Purchase Decisions

Estimated share of different heuristics in an average consumer purchase decision.

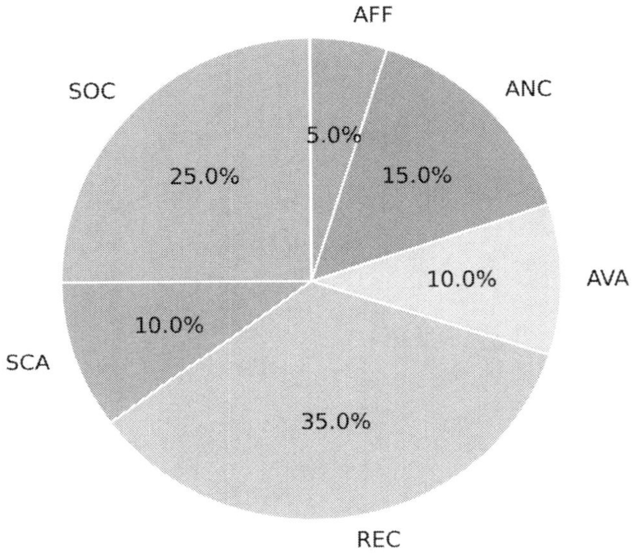

AFF: Affect Heuristic

ANC: Anchoring

AVA: Availability Heuristic

REC: Recognition Heuristic

SCA: Scarcity Heuristic

SOC: Social Proof

The data presented are estimates designed to illustrate the fundamental principles of consumer psychology. They show that a significant portion of purchasing decisions is driven by the Recognition Heuristic (35%) and Social Proof (25%). This suggests that consumers heavily rely on familiar brands and the choices of others, perceiving them as safe and reliable. Anchoring (15%), a common pricing strategy, also plays a substantial role, indicating consumer susceptibility to initial price information. The Availability and Scarcity heuristics (10% each) represent important tactical influences, where recent advertising or perceived limited availability can trigger a purchase. The smallest, yet still relevant, portion is attributed to the Affect Heuristic (5%), highlighting that emotional responses and impulse are also a factor. Overall, the chart visualizes that purchasing decisions are often not purely rational but are strongly shaped by a combination of these mental shortcuts.

5.1.3 Designing Decision Environments for Behavior Guidance

The conscious design of the environment in which decisions are made is an effective tool for steering consumer behavior. This principle, known as decision architecture, posits that the context in which a choice is presented influences the outcome as significantly as the options themselves. Every environment, from the layout of a supermarket to the design of a website, possesses such architecture, which may have arisen randomly or been deliberately conceived to promote specific behaviors. Understanding these mechanisms empowers consumers to recognize subtle attempts at manipulation and enhances their autonomy in the decision-making process.

One of the most effective techniques is the use of defaults (defaults). People tend to stick with the preset option due to convenience or uncertainty. This effect is frequently exploited online, for instance, when a checkbox for newsletter subscription is pre-checked during an order or a more expensive shipping method is selected as the default. The psychological barrier to actively changing a preset is often greater than the perceived benefit of the alternative. To maintain their decision-making authority, it is advisable for consumers to consciously review all options in online forms or configurations and not to interpret the default selection as a neutral recommendation.

The physical arrangement of products in space directs attention and influences the likelihood of selection. In supermarkets, high-margin products are often placed at eye level, while cheaper or specific alternatives are found on lower or upper shelves. This emphasis, referred to as salience, exploits the limited cognitive capacity of shoppers, who rarely scan the entire range systematically. Conversely, prominently placing fruits and vegetables at the entrance of a store can boost sales of these product categories. Consumers can counteract this manipulation by creating a fixed shopping list before shopping and consciously searching less prominent shelf areas.

Such targeted yet subtle interventions in the decision environment are referred to as "nudges." They aim to steer behavior in a predictable direction without prohibiting options or significantly altering economic incentives. A nudge does not formally restrict freedom of choice but makes a particular option the easiest or most obvious choice. This can also affect how information is presented. The structuring of options is an effective means in this regard. If healthy dishes are placed at the beginning of a menu or visually highlighted, their likelihood of selection increases. Another tool is partitioning: large packages of snacks divided into many small, individually wrapped portions slow down consumption, as a new, conscious decision to continue eating must be made after each portion.

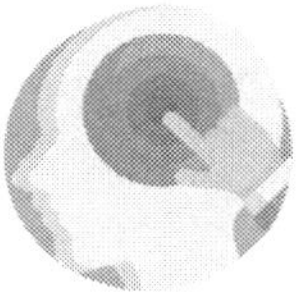

The willingness of retailers to employ such behavior-steering strategies depends on various factors. Social aspects such as customer trust and anticipated consumer needs are crucial for retailers' decision-making. A store will only implement a healthier product arrangement if it believes that customers will accept this offer and not perceive the measure as paternalistic. Consumers who actively seek providers that create positive incentives through transparent and health-promoting environmental design and support these with their purchasing power can shape the offerings in the long term. Thus, the architecture of the decision environment is not a passive backdrop but an active co-creator of purchasing behavior. It interacts directly with the heuristics and cognitive biases previously described by triggering specific mental shortcuts. Analyzing one's shopping environment—whether in a store or on a website—for such designed elements is the first step toward regaining more autonomy in one's decisions.

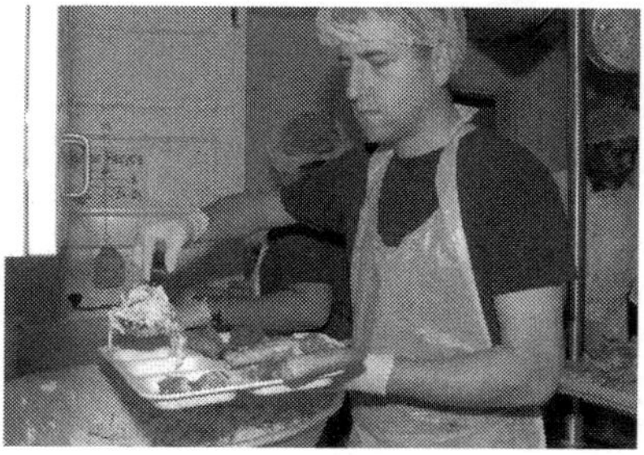

Partitioning [i32]

Good to know

Decision Architecture

Refers to the intentional design of the environment in which a person makes a choice. The goal is to influence the decision through the presentation of options without formally restricting freedom of choice. Every detail, from the order of products to color highlighting, is part of this architecture.

Default

A preset option that automatically applies when no active decision is made. This technique exploits the human tendency toward convenience and the status quo to steer behavior in a specific direction, such as agreeing to newsletters or selecting product variants.

Partitioning

The intentional division of a good into smaller units or portions. This structuring creates artificial interruptions in consumption, each requiring a new, conscious decision. This slows down careless or excessive consumption.

Salience

Describes the property of a stimulus to stand out from its environment and thereby automatically attract attention. In marketing, salience is used to deliberately direct consumer perception toward specific products or information, increasing their likelihood of selection.

Effectiveness of Nudging Techniques

Relative effectiveness of various nudging techniques in influencing consumer choice.

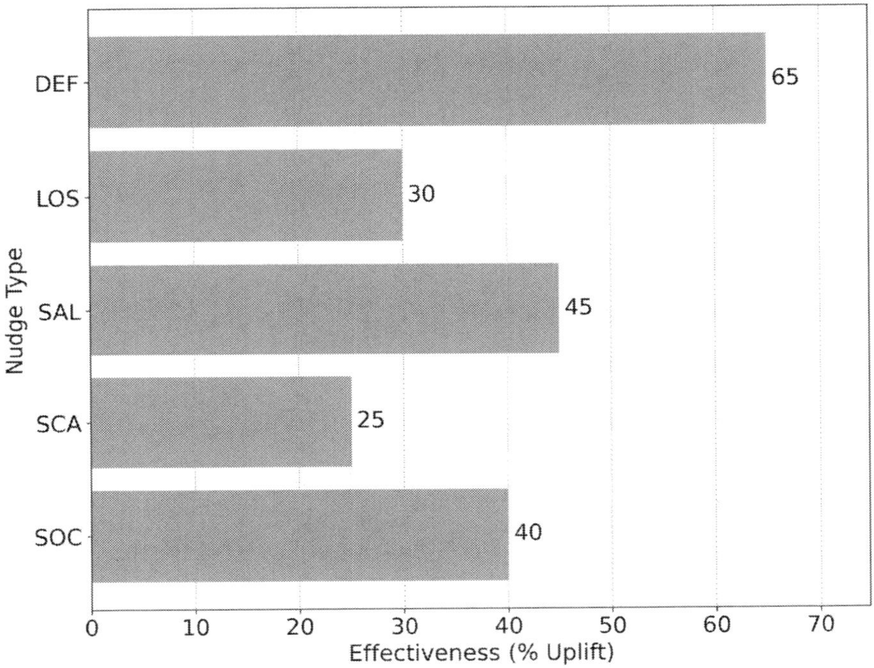

DEF: Default Options

LOS: Loss Aversion

SAL: Salience and Simplicity

SCA: Scarcity

SOC: Social Proof

The chart illustrates the relative impact of different nudging techniques on decision-making. Default settings prove to be the most potent tool, significantly steering choices due to inertia and implied endorsement. Making the desired option simple and prominent (Salience) and leveraging social proof are also highly effective strategies. Techniques like framing choices around potential losses (Loss Aversion) and creating a sense of urgency (Scarcity) show a more moderate, yet still significant, influence. These values are principled estimates intended to illustrate the general hierarchy of effectiveness, as the actual impact can vary greatly depending on the specific context.

Concrete Advice

- Mentally strip a product of its packaging and ask yourself what would remain if it were anonymously placed in a gray box.
- When it comes to discount offers, set your own 'usage anchor' by dividing the price by the estimated number of uses to determine the true value per use.
- Conduct a blind application test with a cheaper alternative for one of your established brand products to separate actual quality from perceived quality.
- Mentally treat free trial periods like a rental and, at the end, ask yourself not 'Do I want to keep it?' but 'Would I pay rent for it again now?'
- Consciously choose the longest checkout line and use the waiting time to check your shopping cart for unnecessary impulse items instead of being tempted by checkout offers.
- Systematically scan supermarket shelves like a book—from the top left to the bottom right—to actively avoid visual guidance at eye level.
- When considering a prominent brand, consciously ask yourself: 'Do I know this product from personal experience or mainly from advertising?' to distinguish pure familiarity from substantiated quality.
- When reading product reviews, specifically focus on the three-star reviews, as these often contain the most balanced critique between blind enthusiasm and pure disappointment.
- Create a list of non-commercial rewards, such as taking a walk or listening to a favorite song, and refer to it when feeling the urge for a 'frustration purchase.'
- Play 'Sales Psychology Bingo' while shopping by actively looking for anchor prices, artificial scarcity, or flattering phrasing.

5. 2 Applying Behavioral Psychology in a Social Context

The gap between good intentions and their implementation is a daily challenge. Pure willpower is rarely sufficient to solidify new habits or permanently shed undesirable behaviors such as procrastination. Often, the crucial role of the social environment as a malleable resource is overlooked. The targeted application of behavioral psychological principles makes a difference here. This chapter illuminates how social reinforcement, conscious learning processes, and a well-founded self-commitment can guide one's actions. It reveals the mechanisms through which the social fabric becomes an effective tool for personal development. The following discussions provide the instruments to systematically and successfully shape one's behavior and social environment.

Sustainable behavioral change does not arise from willpower alone, but through the conscious design of a social environment that reflects and reinforces one's own commitment.

> *Every habit and faculty is confirmed and strengthened by the corresponding actions, that of walking by walking, that of running by running.*

Epictetus

Discourses
Book II, ch. 18, § 1

This statement by Epictetus is a foundational principle of behavioral psychology. It perfectly describes the mechanism of habit formation: behaviors are not innate but are strengthened through repetition. In applied social psychology, this understanding is used to design interventions that encourage positive behaviors—from recycling to healthy eating—by creating contexts and cues that facilitate the repeated practice of the desired action until it becomes automatic.

5.2.1 Building Positive Habits Through Social Reinforcement

Social reinforcement describes the process by which an individual's behavior is shaped by the reactions of their social environment. Positive responses such as praise, recognition, or belonging increase the likelihood that a desired behavior will be repeated. This mechanism can be deliberately utilized to support the establishment of new, positive habits. The human brain is designed to interpret social signals and adjust one's actions accordingly to secure social acceptance and avoid rejection. A new habit, such as regular exercise, is thus reinforced not only by intrinsic motivation or physical effects but also by the positive feedback from friends, family, or a training group.

A fundamental way in which social reinforcement works is through observational learning. People learn behaviors by observing and imitating others, a mechanism described within the social cognitive theory [s33]. When a person sees someone in their environment receiving positive feedback or achieving visible success for a specific behavior, such as consistently adhering to a diet plan, their motivation to adopt that behavior increases. The observed reward acts as a proxy and motivates imitation. Self-efficacy, or the belief in one's ability to accomplish a task, is directly influenced by social support [s33]. Receiving encouragement from others or witnessing individuals with similar circumstances achieve their goals strengthens the conviction that one can succeed as well. A supportive environment thus acts as a catalyst for confidence in one's competencies.

To practically utilize social reinforcement for habit formation, it is effective to consciously shape one's social environment. This means deliberately surrounding oneself with people who already practice the desired behavior or pursue the same goals. Joining a running group, a book club, or an online community for programmers creates a framework where positive behaviors are the norm. Within such groups, a dynamic of mutual motivation and social accountability emerges. The knowledge that others notice one's progress and that one can share successes and setbacks creates a strong external source of motivation.

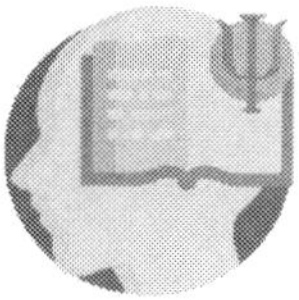

Reinforcement itself can occur in various ways and should be tailored to the specific phase of habit formation. In the initial phase of a new routine, concrete support and encouragement are often helpful. Later, when the habit is already established, recognition of consistency serves as an effective reinforcement. Specifically, this can manifest as sharing one's intention to learn a new skill with a friend. This friend can act as a social reinforcer by regularly inquiring about progress, practicing together, or expressing praise for achieved milestones.

The effectiveness of interventions for behavior change increases when they involve social networks, as this addresses both individual and interpersonal factors simultaneously [s33]. A person trying to quit smoking greatly benefits from a partner or friend group that actively supports this process. This can occur through simple actions, such as avoiding situations that trigger the urge to smoke or celebrating smoke-free weeks together. Social reinforcement manifests here not only through words but also through actions that promote the new, healthy behavior and make the old, undesirable behavior more difficult. By consciously shaping social interactions, the establishment of positive habits transforms from a mere act of will into a collectively supported process.

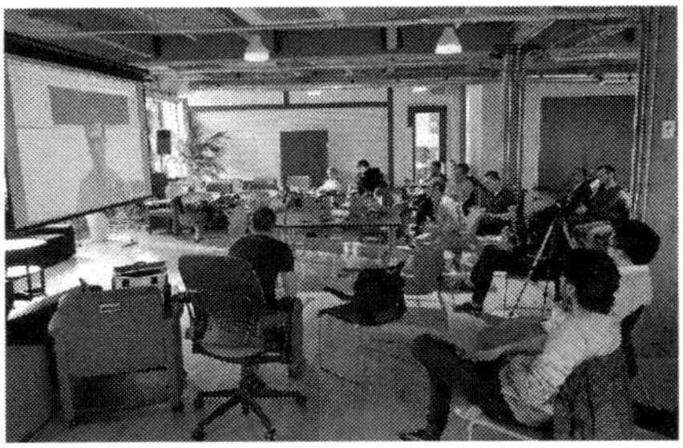

Observational learning [i33]

Good to know

Intrinsic Motivation

The internal drive to perform an action because it is inherently satisfying, interesting, or challenging. In contrast to external rewards, satisfaction lies in the activity itself. An overemphasis on external incentives can even diminish intrinsic motivation.

Social Accountability

The feeling of obligation towards others to follow through on a stated intention. This often arises when goals or intentions are made public, as people strive to be seen as consistent and reliable by others.

Social Cognitive Theory

A theory developed by Albert Bandura that emphasizes that learning occurs in a social interplay. It posits a mutual influence of person, environment, and behavior. Thus, people are not only products of their surroundings but also actively shape them.

Social Reinforcement

Refers to the influence of behavior through social consequences. It can be material (e.g., a gift) or immaterial (e.g., a smile). Particularly effective is irregular reinforcement, as it makes the desired behavior more resilient against the absence of rewards.

Social Reinforcement and Habit Formation

Correlation between the frequency of weekly social reinforcement and the resulting habit strength after a 90-day period.

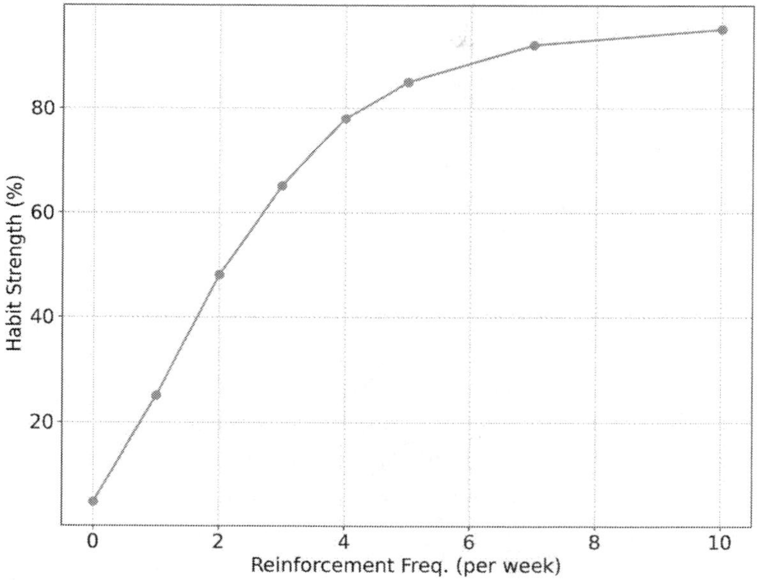

The data illustrates a strong positive correlation between the frequency of social reinforcement and the strength of a new habit. Initially, even a small increase in reinforcement leads to a significant jump in habit strength, highlighting the critical role of early, consistent feedback. As reinforcement becomes more frequent, the habit strength continues to grow, but at a decelerating rate. This pattern suggests a principle of diminishing returns: once a behavior is moderately established, each additional instance of reinforcement provides less incremental benefit. The curve culminates in a plateau, indicating that while frequent social support can build a very strong habit, achieving a fully automated state may depend on other intrinsic factors. These data are principled estimations intended to visually represent the fundamental mechanism of social reinforcement in habit formation.

5.2.2 Application of Learning Principles for Targeted Behavior Change

Learning principles enable a systematic control of behavior changes that go beyond mere conditioning. Instead of merely responding to external rewards or punishments, individuals can learn to actively utilize their social environment as a tool for personal development. This process relies on the conscious design of interactions and group norms to promote desired actions and inhibit unwanted ones. Such an approach is often more effective when based on proven behavioral models, as these provide a framework for understanding why people behave in certain ways and which factors facilitate or block adjustments [s33].

A structured approach to behavior change utilizes the community as a method. This involves not only passive support but also the active establishment of behavioral standards and social accountability within a group [s34]. The community defines clear expectations, and adherence to these norms becomes a driving force for personal growth. The motivation for change derives from both positive incentives, such as recognition from peers, and the gentle pressure created by communal standards. The group acts as a catalyst, maintaining initial motivation and supporting individuals through phases of uncertainty. A collective aiming to overcome procrastination illustrates this. Here, not only is the progress of a member acknowledged, but there is also a collective discussion about why a goal was missed. This form of mutual support, based on honesty and a shared goal of self-improvement, creates an environment where changes can be sustainably anchored [s34].

For such communal processes to take effect, individual skills in self-regulation are necessary. Two techniques are particularly relevant for the individual: clear goal setting and self-monitoring [s33]. Before a behavior change can be successful in a social context, the individual must define for themselves what exactly is to be achieved and how progress will be measured. This lays the foundation for any targeted intervention. Self-monitoring is the mechanism that connects this goal setting with reality. It involves continuously observing and recording one's behavior and is a central component of many successful programs for behavior modification.

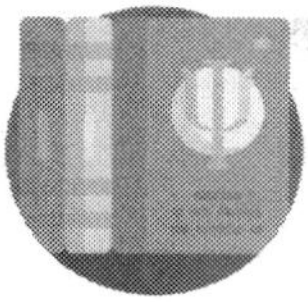

The practical implementation of these principles can be translated into concrete action steps that connect individual self-regulation with the power of the group:

- **Clearly defining the target behavior:** Instead of a vague intention like "live healthier," a specific, measurable goal is formulated, such as "go running three times a week for 30 minutes."
- **Establishing traceable metrics:** Progress is objectively recorded, for example, by keeping a training diary or noting smoke-free days.
- **Regularly documenting one's actions:** This documentation serves not only for control but also makes successes visible and helps identify patterns that lead to setbacks.

These self-monitoring techniques are then introduced into the social context. By sharing goals and progress with a supportive group, a positive social accountability emerges. The group provides not only emotional support but also a structure that holds the individual accountable. The combination of precise self-observation and dynamic interaction within an engaged community creates a robust foundation for lasting behavior change, which would often be unattainable through willpower alone. The intervention thus simultaneously aims to strengthen individual capabilities and create a supportive environment [s33].

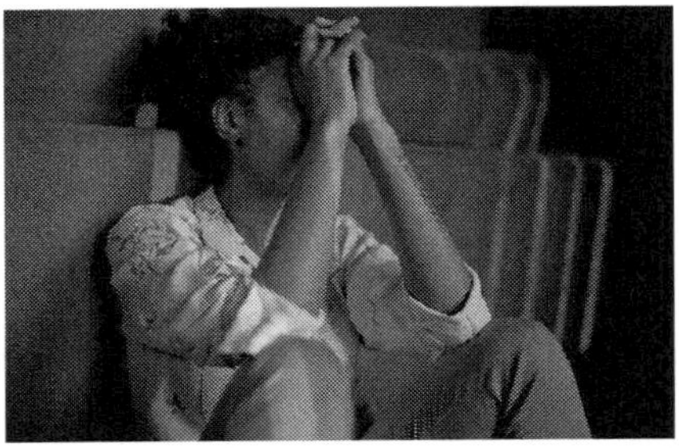

Procrastination [i34]

Good to know

Behavior Modification

An approach based on the principles of learning theory aimed at reducing undesirable behaviors and increasing desirable ones. Techniques such as positive reinforcement through social recognition or systematically ignoring unwanted behavior in a group are employed.

Behavioral Model

Refers to learning through observation and imitation of others. In a social context, individuals often adopt behaviors, attitudes, and emotional responses from role models, especially when these are perceived as successful, likable, or authoritative. This process is a fundamental form of social learning.

Self-Monitoring

A process in which a person directs their attention to their behavior and its effects on others. Individuals with high self-monitoring adapt their behavior significantly to the social situation and the expectations of their counterparts. In contrast, those with low self-monitoring behave more consistently across different situations.

Social Accountability

A psychological state in which a person feels compelled to perform a behavior because they have publicly expressed their intention or stated it to a group. The fear of social devaluation or loss of reputation for failing to meet the promise increases the motivation to pursue the goal.

Principles of Successful Behavior Change

Estimated contribution of different learning principles to successful behavior change.

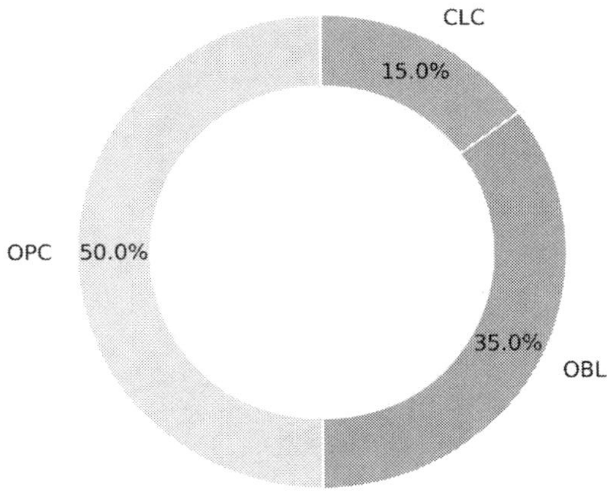

- CLC: Classical Conditioning
- OBL: Observational Learning
- OPC: Operant Conditioning

This distribution illustrates the estimated relative importance of key learning principles in achieving deliberate behavior change. Operant Conditioning, which involves learning through consequences like rewards and punishments, forms the largest share. This underscores its role as a powerful and direct tool for actively shaping new behaviors and habits. Observational Learning holds a significant share, highlighting the immense influence of the social environment. In many situations, we adopt new behaviors by observing role models, peers, and social norms, making this principle crucial for change within a social context. Classical Conditioning, which deals with learning through association (e.g., environmental cues triggering a craving), represents a smaller but fundamental part. It often explains the underlying triggers for old habits, which must be managed for a change to be successful. It is important to note that these figures are conceptual estimates intended to illustrate the general interplay and weight of these principles; in practice, they are often deeply intertwined.

5.2.3 Self-Commitment as a Tool for Sustainable Goal Achievement

Self-commitment is the conscious decision to consistently pursue a specific goal and to carry out the necessary actions. This process resembles a psychological contract with oneself, the stability of which significantly depends on two cognitive evaluations: the perceived significance of the goal (goal significance) and the belief in its attainability (goal attainability). A self-commitment only unfolds its full effect when both aspects are consciously shaped and aligned. It serves as an inner compass that directs actions even when initial motivation wanes or external incentives are lacking.

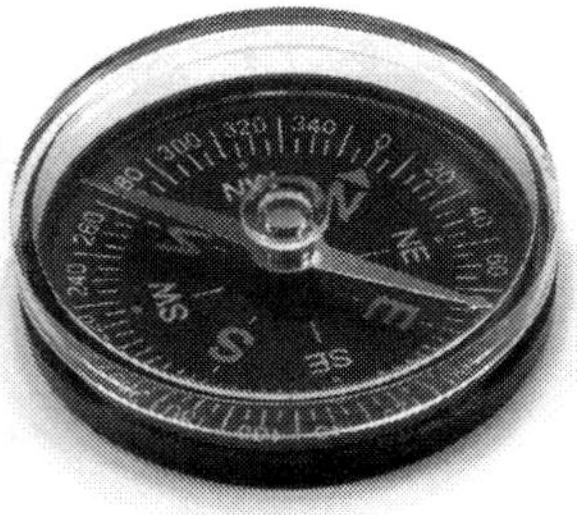

Compass [i35]

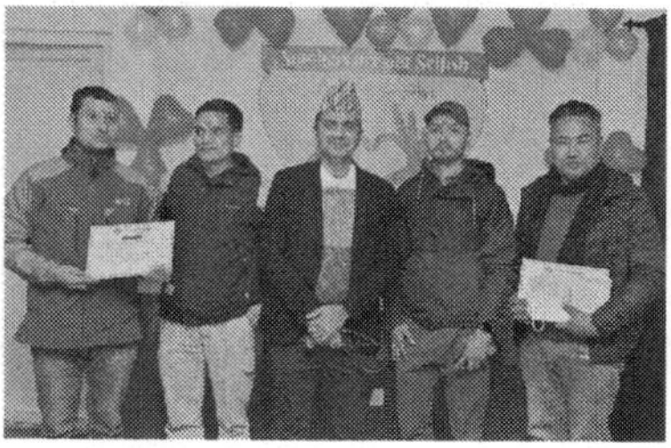

Self-commitment [i36]

The sustainability of a self-commitment is based on the personal relevance of the goal. People commit themselves permanently to endeavors they perceive as meaningful and in alignment with their core values [s19]. An abstract or externally imposed goal, such as "exercising more," often lacks the necessary pull for long-term behavioral change. The real work begins with clarifying the "why." By linking a goal to a profound personal motive, it transforms from a mere task into an expression of one's identity or life planning. An endeavor to save a fixed amount monthly gains strength when it is not just a number but is associated with a deeper personal value—such as the financial security of the family or the realization of a long-held dream. This conscious connection creates an emotional and cognitive bond that serves as a buffer against short-term discomforts or temptations. Motivation then derives not only from the expectation of the end result but also from the process itself, as each action is perceived as a step toward a meaningful state.

Alongside goal significance, perceived attainability must be ensured so that self-commitment does not fail due to unrealistic expectations. A goal perceived as unattainable paralyzes proactive action, even if it is considered very significant [s19]. The art lies in breaking down large, long-term ambitions into a series of concrete, manageable, and measurable steps. This decomposition transforms a vague intention into a clear action plan. The grand goal of purchasing a home is divided into manageable units, for instance, by setting up a standing order for a realistic savings amount immediately after salary receipt. Each successfully completed step strengthens the conviction that the next stage can also be mastered, thereby nourishing the self-efficacy. This process of gradual approach makes progress visible and tangible, which in turn continuously reinforces the self-commitment.

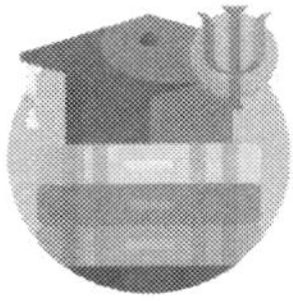

This entire process can be understood as a form of self-leadership, where a person takes on the role of a transformational leader for themselves. They not only define an inspiring vision of the future (goal significance) but also create the structures and conditions that enable successful implementation (goal attainability). In this role, it is about holding oneself accountable without self-condemnation in the face of setbacks. Setbacks are interpreted not as personal failures but as informative deviations from the plan. Instead of abandoning the commitment, the "inner leader" analyzes the causes of the problem—was the step too large, was the timing wrong, or were resources lacking?—and adjusts the strategy. This flexible yet consistent management of one's behavior makes self-commitment a dynamic and resilient tool. It anchors the responsibility for goal achievement internally and creates a stable foundation for lasting changes that persist independently of external control or social applause.

Good to know

Self-Commitment

The effectiveness of a self-commitment can be enhanced by social factors. When a project is made public, social pressure arises that promotes adherence to the commitment, as one's reputation is at stake.

Self-Efficacy

The belief in one's ability to handle difficult social situations or tasks independently. It is strengthened not only by personal successes but also by observing others who master similar challenges.

Transformational

Describes a leadership style aimed at changing the values and goals of followers so that they work for a common goal beyond their own interests. This occurs through inspiration, intellectual stimulation, and individual appreciation.

Effectiveness of Self-Commitment

Success rate of goals based on their difficulty and the type of commitment made.

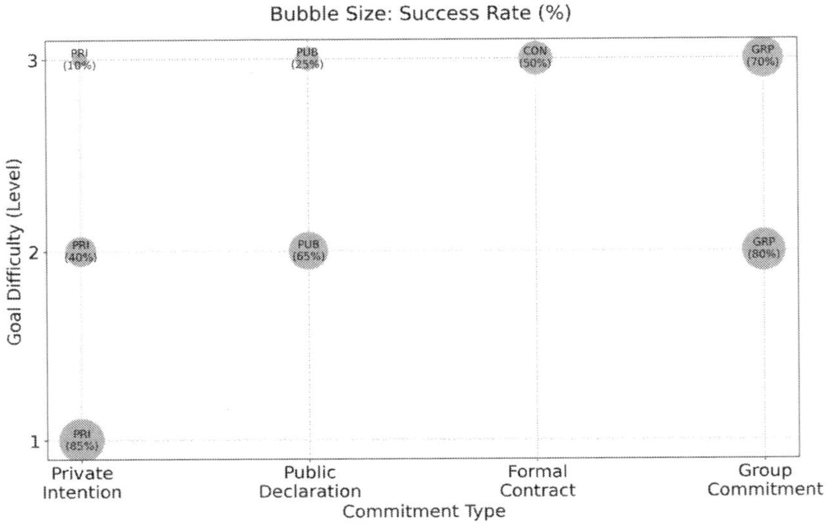

Blasengröße: Success Rate (%)

CON: Formal Contract

GRP: Group Commitment

PRI: Private Intention

PUB: Public Declaration

The chart illustrates a clear correlation between the nature of a commitment, the difficulty of the goal, and the likelihood of success. As goal difficulty (Y-axis) increases, the overall success rate (bubble size) tends to decrease. However, the key insight lies in the impact of the commitment type (X-axis). For any given level of difficulty, a stronger, more socially-binding commitment significantly increases the success rate. The difference is most dramatic for high-difficulty goals: a private, unspoken intention has a very low chance of success, whereas a commitment made within a supportive group context is vastly more effective. This suggests that leveraging social accountability and formal structures is a powerful strategy for achieving challenging, long-term objectives. It is important to note that these data points are estimates designed to illustrate these fundamental principles of behavioral psychology, rather than representing precise statistics from a specific study. They serve to visualize the relative effectiveness of different commitment strategies.

Concrete Advice

- Publicly commit to teaching another person a skill that you do not currently master within a month.
- Form a "Hurdle Alliance" with individuals who want to overcome the same obstacle and agree on a daily, visible proof of successful progress.
- Ask your close circle to actively refer to you by the identity you aspire to, using statements like: "As someone who is now training with discipline, you can do this."
- Establish a "social wager" where you must pay a sum of money to a respected person or complete an unpleasant task for them if you fail to meet your weekly goal.
- Create a fixed transition ritual with a partner, such as a five-minute call right after work, which serves as a social starting signal for the planned evening routine.
- Utilize the principle of reciprocity by doing a significant favor for a friend and merely asking them to hold you accountable for your endeavor in return.
- Make your new habit an attractive, shared experience for your environment, rather than practicing it alone—invite others to cook healthily together instead of just changing your diet.
- Tell a trusted person the story of your success as if you have already achieved your goal, to create a binding emotional reality through verbal narration.
- Create a shared "talisman object" for your group that remains with the member who showed the greatest effort in the previous week, making progress tangible.
- Introduce a "proxy reward" by giving a small gift to a supportive person in your environment for each milestone reached, rather than rewarding yourself.

5.3 Actively Reducing Prejudices and Stereotypes

Prejudices and stereotypes often operate unconsciously. As deeply ingrained thought patterns, they automatically influence our judgments and behaviors in everyday life. These unnoticed influences create social distance, foster misunderstandings, and lead to unfair treatment. This chapter reveals the psychological mechanisms underlying these processes. It demonstrates how such automatism can not only be recognized but also deliberately influenced to promote constructive interactions. The strategies presented provide effective tools to break entrenched thought habits and actively and fairly shape social interactions.

Conscious work on one's own thought patterns is a prerequisite for reducing prejudices, but it is only through the intentional design of positive social interactions that this inner change becomes sustainable and is transformed into lived reality.

> *"It may be doubted whether any character can be named which is distinctive of a race and is constant."*

Charles Darwin

The Descent of Man (1871)
volume I, chapter VII: "On the Races of Man", page 225

Darwin's scientific observation strikes at the very root of stereotyping and racial prejudice. Stereotypes rely on the assumption that fixed, uniform traits can be applied to all members of a group. By highlighting the immense variation within any human population and questioning the existence of constant, distinctive racial characters, Darwin provides a biological and empirical argument against the simplistic and erroneous thinking that underpins prejudice. Reducing prejudice often begins with appreciating this fundamental diversity and challenging the validity of group-based generalizations.

5.3.1 Awareness and Control of Automatic Thought Patterns

Automatic thought patterns are deeply embedded in our cognitive processes. Many stereotypes and prejudices operate unconsciously, influencing our judgment and behavior without our active control. The process of breaking these automatons begins with the awareness of their existence. Implicit prejudices can be compared to mental habits: they have been learned and reinforced over a long time, often unintentionally through societal influences, media, and personal experiences. As with any habit, the first step towards change is to recognize it and develop the motivation to modify it [s35].

Engaging with one's own unconscious associations is not a cause for guilt but rather an objective assessment. Only awareness of one's own prejudices and a genuine concern about their potential discriminatory effects create the necessary internal motivation for change [s35]. External pressure or social expectations prove to be less effective than the self-determined decision to act more justly. Understanding the psychological mechanisms behind prejudices can help address them more openly and less defensively [s36]. The realization that such thought patterns are a normal part of human cognition alleviates pressure and allows for a focus on concrete counter-strategies.

An effective method is individuation, where attention is deliberately directed to the unique characteristics of a person rather than their group membership [s36]. In everyday life, this means consciously detaching from generalizations during encounters. Instead of perceiving a person primarily as a representative of a specific group, one actively focuses on their personal traits, views, and behaviors. One can internally ask questions that shift the focus to the individual: What makes this person unique? What interests do they pursue? What individual experiences shape their perspective? This cognitive act interrupts automatic categorization and promotes a more nuanced perception. Positive emotions during such interactions can support this process, as they reduce the tendency to categorize people primarily by their social or ethnic affiliation [s36].

Another technique is perspective-taking. This involves actively trying to view a situation or issue from another person's perspective. This is more than just empathy; it is the cognitive attempt to see the world through another's eyes and to understand their thoughts and feelings. This exercise can particularly enhance interaction quality in intercultural contexts [s36]. Before judging the behavior of a person from another culture, a brief mental role switch can help. How would the situation appear if one had grown up with that person's cultural norms and life experiences? Such a shift in perspective reduces emotional distance and weakens the basis for stereotypical judgments by emphasizing our common human foundation.

The long-term reduction of prejudices requires the consistent application of such strategies until they become a new habit. This process can be described as active "relearning," where old, problematic associations are replaced by new, conscious, and fair ways of thinking. Research shows that individuals who apply such techniques over several weeks can experience a measurable and lasting reduction in their implicit prejudices [s35]. The strategies can be internalized in a clear sequence to be recalled at critical moments:

- Recognize the stereotype: Notice when a stereotypical thought or prejudice arises.
- Question thoughts: Become aware that it is a generalization and not a fact.
- Replace thoughts: Actively replace the stereotypical thought with a nuanced and individualized consideration.

Through repeated application, this conscious control process becomes increasingly automated. The brain learns to prefer the new, non-stereotypical thought pathways. Thus, the initial effort to control automatic thought patterns gradually transforms into a new, fairer, and more conscious way of perceiving others.

Good to know

Association

A learned, often automatic mental connection between two or more contents, such as a social group and certain characteristics. Stereotypes are based on such established mental links.

Categorization

The fundamental cognitive process of grouping people or objects based on shared characteristics. While this process simplifies thinking, it also forms the basis for the emergence of social stereotypes.

Generalization

The process of inferring from a single case to the general. In the context of stereotypes, this means incorrectly applying a trait observed in a few members of a group to all members of that group.

Individuation

A mental process that counters stereotyping by focusing on the personal and unique information of a person rather than their group membership. This fosters a detailed and less generalized impression.

Perspective-Taking

The conscious effort to understand a situation from the viewpoint of another person. This process can foster empathy, reduce psychological distance to members of other groups, and thus diminish prejudices.

Effectiveness of Bias Reduction Strategies

Estimated relative effectiveness of different techniques to reduce automatic stereotypes.

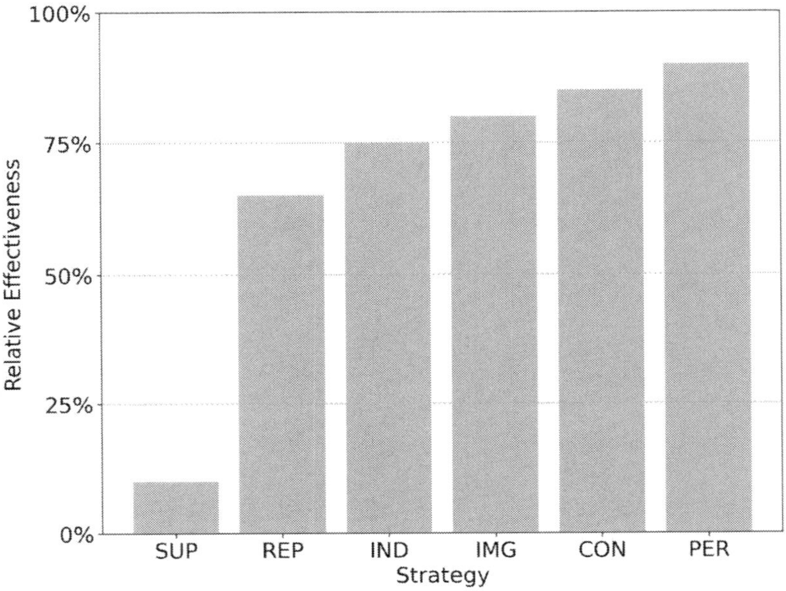

CON: Quality Contact

IND: Individuation

REP: Stereotype Replacement

IMG: Counter-Stereotypic Imaging

PER: Perspective Taking

SUP: Thought Suppression

The chart illustrates that active and engaging strategies are significantly more effective in reducing automatic stereotypes than passive suppression. Techniques like Perspective Taking, which involves actively imagining the experiences of others, and seeking Quality Contact with members of other groups, show the highest effectiveness. In stark contrast, simply trying to suppress stereotypical thoughts is the least effective method and can even be counterproductive, leading to a rebound effect where the stereotypes return stronger. This suggests that a conscious, empathetic, and engaged approach is crucial for successfully breaking down ingrained thought patterns. Please note that the presented values are estimations designed to illustrate the general principles of effectiveness derived from psychological research.

5.3.2 The Design of Positive Intergroup Contact

The conscious engagement with one's own thought patterns is fundamental, yet the reduction of prejudices only fully manifests through direct encounters with individuals from other groups. Mere contact is insufficient and can, if negative, even reinforce stereotypes. Therefore, the intentional design of positive intergroup contact is a crucial step. Social psychology has identified four central conditions that increase the likelihood of a successful, prejudice-reducing exchange. When these conditions are considered in encounter situations, they can sustainably change the way we perceive members of other groups.

A fundamental prerequisite is the equal status of the individuals involved in the contact situation. When members of different groups interact on equal footing, rather than in hierarchical or dependent roles, a basis for mutual respect is established. Unequal power dynamics, such as those present in a supervisor-employee relationship or in helping and receiving help roles, can inadvertently confirm existing stereotypes about the competence and status of groups. Positive contact is more likely to occur in situations where everyone acts as an equal partner. This can be actively promoted by engaging in clubs, shared hobby groups, or neighborhood initiatives, where a common passion or shared goal diminishes group membership and brings everyone together as equal participants.

The second condition is shared goals. When groups must collaborate to achieve a goal that neither group can accomplish alone, a functional necessity for cooperation arises. This interdependence leads to the blurring of rigid boundaries between "us" and "them." A new, overarching sense of "we" emerges. In practice, this could involve jointly organizing a neighborhood festival, working in a mixed project team to solve a specific problem, or participating in a team sport. The focus shifts from the differences between the groups to the collective efforts that lead to success. Every contribution is recognized as valuable for the overall outcome, regardless of the individual's background.

This directly leads to the third condition: intergroup cooperation. Contact should not only occur side by side but should involve active, joint action. Passive contact, such as merely living in the same neighborhood without real interaction, shows minimal effects. Only cooperative collaboration on the previously mentioned shared goals makes contact effective. Through collaboration, individuals come to know each other as unique individuals with specific skills, ideas, and personalities. These personal experiences gradually replace the abstract and often negative stereotypes held about the entire group.

Finally, support from authorities, laws, or social norms is beneficial for the effectiveness of intergroup contact. When leaders in organizations, teachers in schools, or public administration clearly signal that they advocate for positive relationships between different groups and reject discrimination, this creates an atmosphere of safety and legitimacy. This institutional support encourages individuals to approach others more openly while simultaneously sanctioning negative, exclusionary behavior.

The effects of high-quality contact are profound. Studies show that adolescents from ethnic minorities who have regular and positive contact with members of the majority society are more likely to recognize and condemn racially motivated exclusion as unjust [s37]. They develop a better understanding of how stereotypes are used by others to justify exclusion. In contrast, individuals with little intergroup contact often feel insecure and do not know how to respond to discriminatory situations [s37]. Positive contact thus not only conveys a more nuanced image of others but also strengthens one's competence to advocate for fairness and against exclusion. Through repeated experiences that cooperation and exchange yield positive outcomes for all, a fundamental attitude based on openness and mutual recognition is fostered.

Good to know

Discrimination

Represents the behavioral component of prejudice. It is the unjustified negative or harmful action towards an individual based solely on their membership in a particular group.

Interdependence

Describes the mutual dependence of group members in achieving a goal. A well-known application is the 'Jigsaw Method,' where each person possesses a unique part of knowledge that the group needs for success. This makes every contribution indispensable.

Intergroup Contact

Refers to the encounter between members of various social groups. Successful contact relies not only on direct interaction but also reduces the fear and uncertainty that individuals often feel when dealing with out-groups, leading to a more open attitude.

Intergroup Cooperation

Refers to the active collaboration between members of different groups. This process promotes the so-called recategorization, where the boundaries between the original groups blur and a new, shared group identity emerges.

Factors for Successful Prejudice Reduction

Estimated contribution of different conditions to the effectiveness of intergroup contact in reducing prejudice.

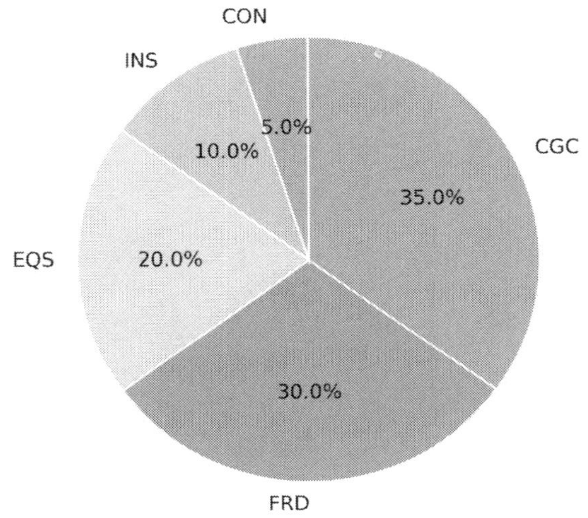

CGC: Cooperation on Common Goals
CON: Mere Contact (Unstructured)
EQS: Equal Status between Groups
FRD: Development of Friendships
INS: Institutional Support

This chart illustrates the estimated relative importance of key conditions for successfully reducing prejudice through intergroup contact. It is important to note that these figures are estimates designed to represent general principles derived from decades of social psychological research. The chart clearly shows that 'Cooperation on Common Goals' and the 'Development of Friendships' are the most powerful drivers, accounting for a significant portion of the positive effect. This underscores that passive, unstructured contact is far less effective than active, goal-oriented collaboration that fosters personal bonds. 'Equal Status' serves as a critical foundation, without which contact can reinforce existing hierarchies and stereotypes. While 'Institutional Support' has a smaller direct share, it is a crucial enabling factor that creates a supportive environment for the other conditions to flourish. The minimal impact of 'Mere Contact' highlights the core message: it is the quality and structure of contact, not just its occurrence, that leads to meaningful and lasting prejudice reduction.

5.3.3 Creation of Common Superordinate Identities

Building on the cooperative collaboration that generates an initial sense of "we," the reduction of prejudices can be further deepened through the deliberate creation of common, superordinate identities. This approach of recategorization aims to redraw the mental boundaries between an in-group ("we") and an out-group ("them"). Instead of perceiving individuals primarily based on distinguishing characteristics such as origin, department, or social affiliation, the focus shifts to a broader, shared identity that includes all parties involved. The previously separate groups thus become subgroups of a new, larger entity. The fundamental psychological principle behind this is that the positive perceptions and cooperative behaviors we typically extend to members of our own group are transferred to members of the former out-group as soon as they become part of the new, expanded "we."

In practice, this means actively seeking and emphasizing commonalities. In a neighborhood with long-standing and newly arrived residents, the focus could shift away from this division and towards a shared identity as "neighbors of the neighborhood," who work together for the safety and cleanliness of their area. This new common identity does not erase previous group affiliations, but they lose relevance for everyday interaction. The perception shifts from "the long-standing residents" versus "the newcomers" to "all of us who live here and want a pleasant environment." The former out-group is now seen as part of the solution to a common concern.

An evolution of this approach is the model of dual identity. This approach posits that prejudices are particularly effectively reduced when both the original group affiliation is maintained and a new, common identity is created [s38]. It is not about blurring or replacing existing identities, but rather establishing an additional, superordinate level of identity. The recognition of subgroup identity signals appreciation and prevents members of a group from feeling assimilated or threatened by the superordinate identity assimilation. This promotes their willingness to embrace the common identity. The simultaneous emphasis on the common identity directs focus to the connections and the necessity for cooperation.

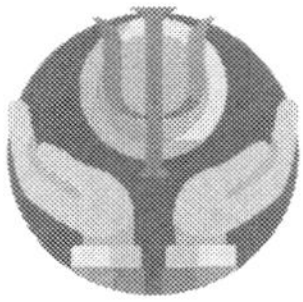

This model can be purposefully applied in everyday life. A team leader in a multinational company can consciously highlight the different cultural backgrounds and professional expertise of team members as valuable resources for creative solutions (recognition of subgroups) while simultaneously emphasizing the team's common mission and belonging to the company as a unifying element (creation of the superordinate identity). The message here is: "Our different perspectives make us strong as a team, and as a team, we work together towards our goal." This dual emphasis can maximize the positive effects of contact, as it satisfies both the need for individual recognition and the need for shared belonging [s38]. The psychological distance decreases without individuals feeling they must give up part of their personal or cultural identity. Instead, a more complex and inclusive identity structure emerges, based on the coexistence of differences within a common framework.

Good to know

In-group

Refers to the group to which an individual feels they belong and whose members they tend to prefer and evaluate more positively than members of other groups.

Model of Dual Identity

An approach that seeks to enhance the positive effects of contact between groups by simultaneously addressing the human need for uniqueness (through the maintenance of subgroup identity) and the need for belonging (through the establishment of superordinate identity).

Out-group

A social group from which a person distances themselves and to which they do not feel they belong. The perception of an out-group is often associated with more negative evaluations and stereotypical notions.

Recategorization

A mental process in which the perception of separate groups (e.g., 'Department A' and 'Department B') is replaced by emphasizing a common belonging (e.g., 'our company'). This promotes the application of positive in-group characteristics to the former out-group.

Subgroup Identity

Refers to the sense of belonging to an original group that continues to exist and is recognized as valuable even after the creation of a common, superordinate identity.

Superordinate Identity and Bias Reduction

Correlation between the strength of a common superordinate identity and the level of intergroup bias.

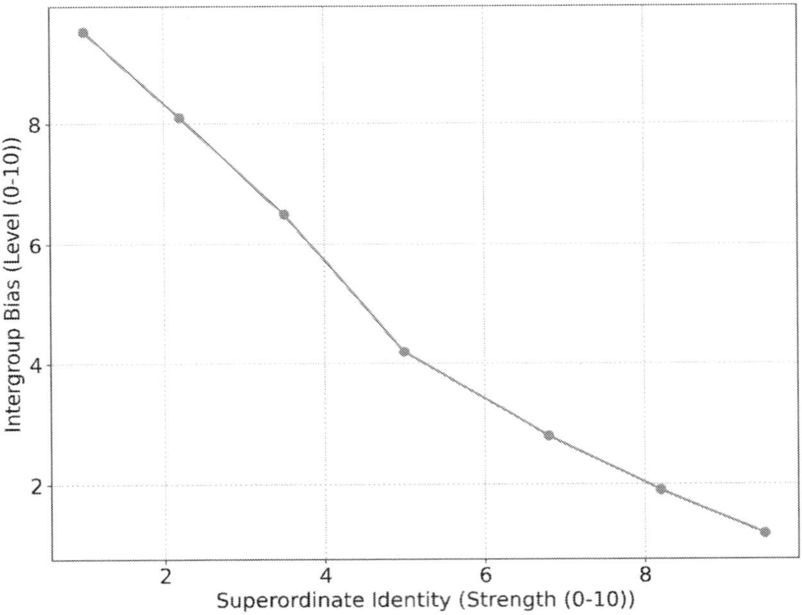

The data illustrates a strong negative correlation: as the perceived strength of a common, superordinate identity increases, the level of bias between groups decreases significantly. The most substantial reduction in bias occurs during the initial formation of a shared identity. Further strengthening this common identity continues to reduce prejudice, although the effect becomes more gradual. This pattern suggests that fostering a sense of a shared 'we' is a highly effective strategy for overcoming intergroup divisions. It is important to note that these data points are illustrative estimates designed to represent the fundamental principle of the 'Common Ingroup Identity Model' from social psychology, showcasing the typical inverse relationship between the strength of a shared identity and the level of intergroup bias.

Concrete Advice

- Invent a brief, complex fictional life story in your mind for a person you are tempted to categorize, in order to replace a one-dimensional perception with a multifaceted one.
- Actively seek out films or books that depict members of a group in atypical, complex roles to enrich your inner imaginative space with new images.
- In conversations with people from other groups, specifically inquire about their daily routines or small joys to discover the common human foundation in the mundane.
- Mentally declare every person who contradicts a stereotype not as an exception, but as the first evidence of the invalidity of the entire rule.
- Pay attention to your own language and consistently replace blanket group labels like "the politicians" with more precise formulations such as "some representatives of this party."
- Deconstruct a stereotypical joke you hear like a riddle: What outdated assumption does it rely on, and whose perspective does it render invisible?
- Actively seek a role model from a group you have previously approached with prejudice and analyze which specific qualities you admire in that person.
- When a stereotypical assumption arises, engage in an internal dialogue where you confront that assumption with "Why?" questions until it breaks down into its components.
- Create a conscious, positive experience by deliberately consuming a product, service, or artwork from a person belonging to a group unfamiliar to you.

Review - 5. Applied Social Psychology: Consumer and Behavior Control in Everyday Life

The social psychological insights into consumption and behavior control reveal an everyday reality in which we act far less autonomously than we often assume. Daily, we navigate an invisible web of advertising messages, cleverly designed environments, and psychological incentives that subtly yet effectively steer our decisions. The first and crucial step towards regaining your agency lies not in resisting individual temptations but in consciously perceiving these mechanisms. Recognize the emotional appeal behind a brand to which you are loyal, or the artificially created time pressure of a "valid only today" offer for what they are: targeted strategies aimed at the efficient yet vulnerable shortcuts of our brains. This awareness is not an admission of weakness but the activation of your rational control instance and the foundation for any conscious behavioral change.

To actively confront this control in everyday life, practical counter-strategies are needed that you can employ as mental tools. Implement a personal 24-hour rule before making significant purchases: place the product in your virtual shopping cart or leave it in the store and give yourself a day to think it over. This simple delay breaks the cycle of emotional impulse and immediate reward triggered by scarcity signals or clever framing. Make it a habit not only to write a shopping list before entering a supermarket but to view it as a binding action plan. This not only protects you from impulse buys at the checkout but also from the strategic placement of products at eye level. Challenge yourself to consciously inspect the less popular shelf space at the bottom or the very top—often, better rational alternatives are hidden there. These small behavioral changes act like a cognitive shield against the automated processes that marketing knows how to exploit so masterfully.

The greatest challenge in implementing these recommendations lies in the omnipresence of stimuli and the limited capacity of our willpower. It is unrealistic and exhausting to subject every single purchasing decision to in-depth analysis. Therefore, focus your energy strategically: apply the techniques primarily to decisions that have a greater financial or long-term impact. For everyday small matters, it is more helpful to proactively shape your environment. If you know that you are prone to unhealthy snacks after a stressful day, ensure that healthy alternatives are more accessible. Recognize patterns in your behavior—do you often shop online when you are bored?—and develop alternative, constructive habits for those moments, such as a brief phone call with a friend or reading a few pages of a book. This is not about deprivation but about directing the satisfaction of a need in a way that serves your long-term goals.

Ultimately, engaging with applied social psychology in the context of consumption is an invitation to self-leadership. It empowers you to shape the architecture of your decisions rather than passively accepting them. By learning to identify the psychological triggers in your environment and consciously managing your reactions to them, you transform from a consumer driven by external forces into a self-determined architect of your daily life. This path does not lead to a life free from influence, but to one in which your actions increasingly align with your true values and goals—a rewarding form of personal autonomy.

Free Additional Offers Planned

We are pleased to offer you free supplementary materials for this book in the future:

- An exclusive bonus chapter with additional content
- A compact summary of the entire book in PDF format
- An audiobook version (In Planning)

These materials are expected to be released in 2025.

www.SaageBooks.com/social_psychology-bonus-VUR6ZN

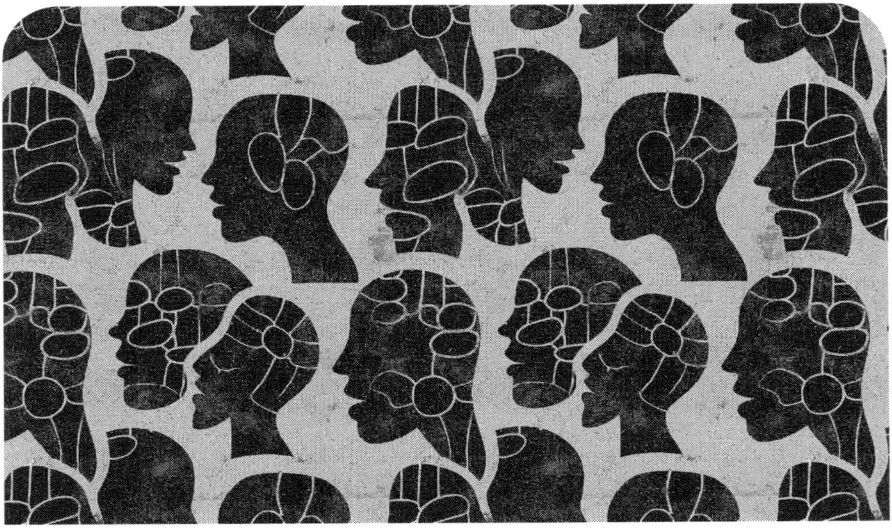

Dear readers,

We are deeply honored that you have taken the time to read our book from beginning to end. Our greatest wish is to provide you with valuable insights and practical guidance. Your trust in our work means a lot to us. We hope the reading was enriching for you. If you have any questions or suggestions, please feel free to contact us through our website.

We would greatly appreciate an honest review. You can easily leave your honest rating on the sales platform where you purchased the book.
Thank you for your support!

Donar A.I. Saage

Saage Media GmbH - Team

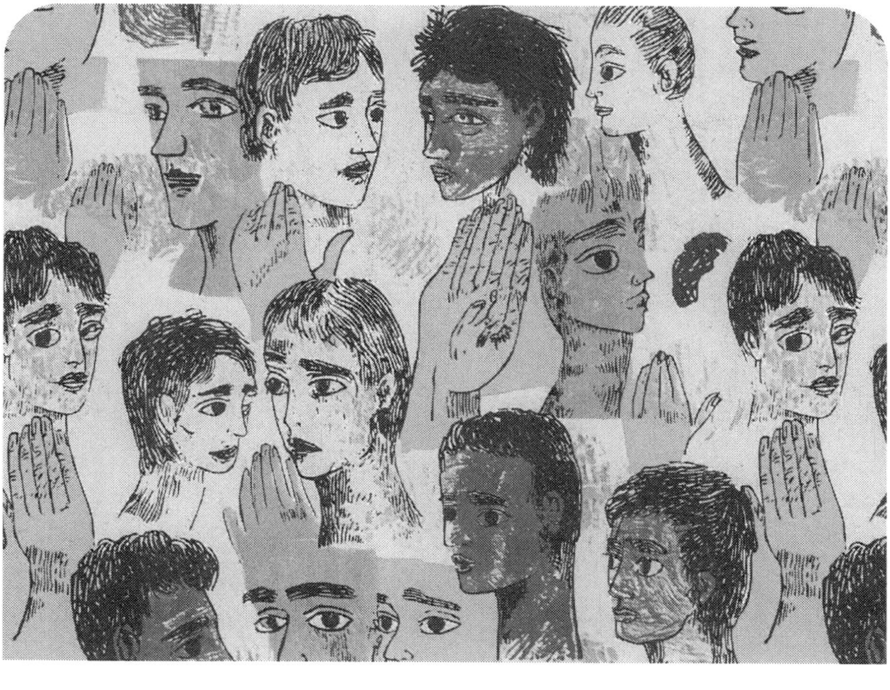

Sources

Our sincere thanks go to all authors of the cited scientific and non-scientific sources, the operators of the referenced websites, and the creators of the images, graphics, and studies used, whose valuable work has contributed to the creation of this book.

For more information, we recommend visiting the source websites.

If you discover any mapping errors or other inconsistencies, please contact us.

All sources were last accessed on: 2025-07-03

[s1] - https://pmc.ncbi.nlm.nih.gov/articles/PMC11276240/

Author:	Mariana Merino (Faculty of Sports Sciences, Universidad Europea de Madrid, 28670 Madrid, Spain); José Francisco Tornero-Aguilera (Faculty of Sports Sciences, Universidad Europea de Madrid, 28670 Madrid, Spain); Alejandro Rubio-Zarapuz (Faculty of Sports Sciences, Universidad Europea de Madrid, 28670 Madrid, Spain); Carlota Valeria Villanueva-Tobaldo (Faculty of Biomedical and Health Sciences, Universidad Europea de Madrid, 28670 Madrid, Spain); Alexandra Martín-Rodríguez (Faculty of Sports Sciences, Universidad Europea de Madrid, 28670 Madrid, Spain); Vicente Javier Clemente-Suárez (Faculty of Sports Sciences, Universidad Europea de Madrid, 28670 Madrid, Spain; Grupo de Investigación en Cultura, Educación y Sociedad, Universidad de la Costa, Barranquilla 080002, Colombia)	**Title:**	Body Perceptions and Psychological Well-Being: A Review of the Impact of Social Media and Physical Measurements on Self-Esteem and Mental Health with a Focus on Body Image Satisfaction and Its Relationship with Cultural and Gender Factors
DOI:	10.3390/healthcare12141396	**Date:**	2024 Jul 12
Website:	PubMed Central (PMC)	**Publisher:**	Healthcare

[s2] - https://pmc.ncbi.nlm.nih.gov/articles/PMC8564255/

Author:	Nexhmedin Morina (Institute of Psychology, University of Münster)	**Title:**	Comparisons Inform Me Who I Am: A General Comparative-Processing Model of Self-Perception
DOI:	10.1177/1745691620966788	**Date:**	2021 Feb 22
Website:	PubMed Central (PMC)	**Publisher:**	National Center for Biotechnology Information (NCBI), National Library of Medicine (NLM), National Institutes of Health (NIH)

[s3] - https://pmc.ncbi.nlm.nih.gov/articles/PMC10943642/

Author:	Rocco Servidio (Department of Culture, Education and Society, University of Calabria, Via Pietro Bucci, Building Cube 20/B, 87036 Arcavacata di Rende, Cosenza, Italy) Paolo Soraci (Università Niccolo Cusano, Via Don Carlo Gnocchi, n.3, Roma, Italy)Mark D Griffiths (International Gaming Research Unit, Psychology Department, Nottingham Trent University, Nottingham, United Kingdom)Stefano Boca (Department of Psychology, Educational Science and Human Movement, University of Palermo, 90128 Palermo, Italy)Zsolt Demetrovics (Centre of Excellence in Responsible Gaming, University of Gibraltar, Gibraltar, Gibraltar, Spain; Institute of Psychology, ELTE Eötvös Loránd University, Budapest, Hungary)	**Title:**	Fear of missing out and problematic social media use: A serial mediation model of social comparison and self-esteem
by:	National Library of Medicine (NLM)	**DOI:**	10.1016/j.abrep.2024.100536
Date:	2024 Mar 5	**Website:**	PubMed Central (PMC)
Publisher:	Elsevier		

[s4] - https://pmc.ncbi.nlm.nih.gov/articles/PMC10080933/

Title:	How photo editing in social media shapes self-perceived attractiveness and self-esteem via self-objectification and physical appearance comparisons	**by:**	Ruhr-Universität Bochum
DOI:	10.1186/s40359-023-01143-0	**Date:**	2023 Apr 6
Website:	PubMed Central (PMC)	**Publisher:**	BMC Psychology

[s5] - https://pmc.ncbi.nlm.nih.gov/articles/PMC6667174/

Title:	The Development of Self and Identity in Adolescence: Neural Evidence and Implications for a Value-Based Choice Perspective on Motivated Behavior	**by:**	University of Oregon
DOI:	10.1111/cdep.12279	**Date:**	2018 Feb 8
Website:	PubMed Central (PMC)	**Publisher:**	National Library of Medicine (NLM), National Institutes of Health (NIH)

[s6] - https://pmc.ncbi.nlm.nih.gov/articles/PMC6258780/

Title:	Personal Branding: Interdisciplinary Systematic Review and Research Agenda	**by:**	Vrije Universiteit Amsterdam
DOI:	10.3389/fpsyg.2018.02238	**Date:**	2018 Nov 21
Website:	PubMed Central (PMC)	**Publisher:**	Frontiers Media SA

[s7] - https://pmc.ncbi.nlm.nih.gov/articles/PMC11794495/

Author:	Daniel Zimmermann, Department of Psychology, University of Cologne, Cologne, Germany; Colleen Schneider, Department of Psychology, University of Cologne, Cologne, Germany; Kai Kaspar, Department of Psychology, University of Cologne, Cologne, Germany	**Title:**	A mixed methods exploration of self-presentation, authenticity, and role model function on Instagram: perspectives from female influencers in Germany
DOI:	10.3389/fpsyg.2024.1472514	**Date:**	2025 Jan 22
Website:	PubMed Central (PMC)	**Publisher:**	National Library of Medicine (NLM)

[s8] - https://pmc.ncbi.nlm.nih.gov/articles/PMC7217460/

Author:	Wangshuai Wang, School of Management, Shanghai University of International Business and Economics, Shanghai, People's Republic of China; Ke Zhou, Antai College of Economics and Management, Shanghai Jiao Tong University, Shanghai, People's Republic of China; Zucheng Yu, School of International Relations and Public Affairs, Shanghai International Studies University, Shanghai, People's Republic of China; Jie Li, School of Management, Shanghai University, Shanghai, People's Republic of China	**Title:**	The Cost of Impression Management to Life Satisfaction: Sense of Control and Loneliness as Mediators
DOI:	10.2147/PRBM.S238344	**Date:**	2020 May 8
Website:	PubMed Central (PMC)	**Publisher:**	Dove Medical Press

[s9] - https://pmc.ncbi.nlm.nih.gov/articles/PMC7686841/

Author:	Sebastian Cancino-Montecinos (Division of Personality, Social, and Developmental Psychology, Department of Psychology, Stockholm University, Stockholm, Sweden); Fredrik Björklund (Division of Personality and Social Psychology, Department of Psychology, Lund University, Lund, Sweden); Torun Lindholm (Division of Personality, Social, and Developmental Psychology, Department of Psychology, Stockholm University, Stockholm, Sweden)	**Title:**	A General Model of Dissonance Reduction: Unifying Past Accounts via an Emotion Regulation Perspective
DOI:	10.3389/fpsyg.2020.540081	**Date:**	2020 Nov 11
Website:	PubMed Central (PMC)	**Publisher:**	National Center for Biotechnology Information (NCBI)

[s10] - https://pmc.ncbi.nlm.nih.gov/articles/PMC4780412/

Author:	Dolores Albarracín (University of Florida), Joel B Cohen (University of Florida), G Tarcan Kumkale (University of Florida)	**Title:**	When Communications Collide With Recipients' Actions: Effects of Post-Message Behavior on Intentions to Follow the Message Recommendation
DOI:	10.1177/0146167203029007003	**Date:**	2003 Jul
Website:	PubMed Central (PMC)	**Publisher:**	SAGE Publications

[s11] - https://pmc.ncbi.nlm.nih.gov/articles/PMC8657395/

Author:	Rui Shi, Department of Communication Studies, Ric Edelman College of Communication & Creative Arts, Rowan University, Glassboro, New Jersey, USA; Jiaying Liu, Department of Communication Studies, University of Georgia, Athens, Georgia, USA; Joseph N Cappella, Annenberg School for Communication, University of Pennsylvania, Philadelphia, Pennsylvania, USA	**Title:**	Influence of Online Comments on Smokers' E-cigarette Attitude: Opinion Climate, Review Fraud, and Resistance to Persuasion
DOI:	10.1080/08870446.2021.1893320	**Date:**	2021 Mar 15
Website:	PubMed Central (PMC)	**Publisher:**	National Library of Medicine (NLM)

[s12] - https://pmc.ncbi.nlm.nih.gov/articles/PMC11420015/

Author:	Lichao Xiu (Laboratory of Cognitive Neuroscience and Communication, School of Journalism and Communication, Beijing Normal University, Beijing, China)Xuejiao Chen (Laboratory of Cognitive Neuroscience and Communication, School of Journalism and Communication, Beijing Normal University, Beijing, China)Lulu Mao (Laboratory of Cognitive Neuroscience and Communication, School of Journalism and Communication, Beijing Normal University, Beijing, China)Enyu Zhang (Laboratory of Cognitive Neuroscience and Communication, School of Journalism and Communication, Beijing Normal University, Beijing, China)Guoming Yu (Laboratory of Cognitive Neuroscience and Communication, School of Journalism and Communication, Beijing Normal University, Beijing, China)	**Title:**	Unveiling the influence of persuasion strategies on cognitive engagement: an ERPs study on attentional search
DOI:	10.3389/fnbeh.2024.1302770	**Date:**	2024 Sep 10
Website:	PubMed Central (PMC)	**Publisher:**	Frontiers Media SA

[s13] - https://pmc.ncbi.nlm.nih.gov/articles/PMC8653370/

Author:	Han Zheng (Wee Kim Wee School of Communication and Information, Nanyang Technological University, Singapore); Dion Hoe-Lian Goh (Wee Kim Wee School of Communication and Information, Nanyang Technological University, Singapore); Edmund Wei Jian Lee (Wee Kim Wee School of Communication and Information, Nanyang Technological University, Singapore); Chei Sian Lee (Wee Kim Wee School of Communication and Information, Nanyang Technological University, Singapore); Yin-Leng Theng (Wee Kim Wee School of Communication and Information, Nanyang Technological University, Singapore)	**Title:**	Understanding the effects of message cues on COVID-19 information sharing on Twitter
DOI:	10.1002/asi.24587	**Date:**	2021 Oct 15
Website:	PubMed Central (PMC)	**Publisher:**	Journal of the Association for Information Science and Technology

[s14] - https://pmc.ncbi.nlm.nih.gov/articles/PMC2779518/

Title:	Age Differences in Resistance to Peer Influence	**by:**	National Library of Medicine (NLM)
DOI:	10.1037/0012-1649.43.6.1531	**Date:**	2007 Nov
Website:	PubMed Central (PMC)	**Publisher:**	National Library of Medicine

[s15] - https://pmc.ncbi.nlm.nih.gov/articles/PMC10008044/

Author:	Dušan Mladenović (Department of Business Management, Faculty of Economics and Administration, Masaryk University, Brno, Czech Republic); Michal Jirásek (Department of Business Management, Faculty of Economics and Administration, Masaryk University, Brno, Czech Republic); Tomáš Ondrá ček (Department of Business Management, Faculty of Economics and Administration, Masaryk University, Brno, Czech Republic); Zuzana Opatrná (Department of Business Management, Faculty of Economics and Administration, Masaryk University, Brno, Czech Republic); Radmila Štangová (Department of Business Management, Faculty of Economics and Administration, Masaryk University, Brno, Czech Republic)	**Title:**	The influence of social conformity on mask-wearing behavior during the COVID-19 pandemic
by:	Masaryk University	**DOI:**	10.1016/j.heliyon.2023.e14496
Date:	2023 Mar 11	**Website:**	PubMed Central (PMC)
Publisher:	Elsevier		

[s16] - https://pmc.ncbi.nlm.nih.gov/articles/PMC5931497/

Author:	Daniel J Mallinson, Peter K Hatemi	**Title:**	The effects of information and social conformity on opinion change
by:	National Library of Medicine (NLM)	**DOI:**	10.1371/journal.pone.0196600
Date:	2018 May 2	**Website:**	PubMed Central (PMC)
Publisher:	PLoS ONE		

[s17] - https://pmc.ncbi.nlm.nih.gov/articles/PMC8617051/

Author:	Emilie A Caspar	**Title:**	A novel experimental approach to study disobedience to authority
DOI:	10.1038/s41598-021-02334-8	**Date:**	2021 Nov 25
Website:	PubMed Central (PMC)		

[s18] - https://pmc.ncbi.nlm.nih.gov/articles/PMC3460209/
Author: Sara A Kreindler (Winnipeg Regional Health Authority, University of Manitoba); Damien A Dowd (Winnipeg Regional Health Authority, University of Manitoba); Noah Dana Star (Winnipeg Regional Health Authority, University of Winnipeg); Tania Gottschalk (University of Manitoba)
Title: Silos and Social Identity: The Social Identity Approach as a Framework for Understanding and Overcoming Divisions in Health Care
DOI: 10.1111/j.1468-0009.2012.00666.x
Date: 2012 Jun 18
Website: PubMed Central (PMC)
Publisher: The Milbank Quarterly

[s19] - https://pmc.ncbi.nlm.nih.gov/articles/PMC6281759/
Title: The Path Is the Goal: How Transformational Leaders Enhance Followers' Job Attitudes and Proactive Behavior
by: Bielefeld University
DOI: 10.3389/fpsyg.2018.02338
Date: 2018 Nov 29
Website: PubMed Central (PMC)
Publisher: Frontiers in Psychology

[s20] - https://pmc.ncbi.nlm.nih.gov/articles/PMC8157163/
Title: "Despite the Differences, We Were All the Same". Group Cohesion in Diagnosis-Specific and Transdiagnostic CBT Groups for Anxiety and Depression: A Qualitative Study
by: National Center for Biotechnology Information (NCBI)
DOI: 10.3390/ijerph18105324
Date: 2021-05-17
Website: PubMed Central (PMC)

[s21] - https://pmc.ncbi.nlm.nih.gov/articles/PMC6374220/
Author: Manon A van Scheppingen (University of Amsterdam, Amsterdam, Netherlands); William J Chopik (Michigan State University, East Lansing, United States); Wiebke Bleidorn (University of California, Davis, United States); Jaap JA Denissen (Tilburg University, Tilburg, Netherlands)
Title: Longitudinal Actor, Partner and Similarity Effects of Personality on Well-Being
DOI: 10.1037/pspp0000211
Date: 2018 Aug 13
Website: PubMed Central (PMC)
Publisher: American Psychological Association (APA)

[s22] - https://pubmed.ncbi.nlm.nih.gov/5660731/
Author: Byrne D;London O;Reeves K;
Title: The effects of physical attractiveness, sex, and attitude similarity on interpersonal attraction
DOI: 10.1111/j.1467-6494.1968.tb01473.x
Date: 1968 Jun
Website: PubMed
Publisher: Journal of personality

[s23] - https://pmc.ncbi.nlm.nih.gov/articles/PMC2811283/

Author:	Leslie A Zebrowitz (Brandeis University), Joann M Montepare (Emerson College)	**Title:**	Social Psychological Face Perception: Why Appearance Matters
DOI:	10.1111/j.1751-9004.2008.00109.x	**Date:**	2008 May 1
Website:	PubMed Central (PMC)	**Publisher:**	Wiley-Blackwell

[s24] - https://pmc.ncbi.nlm.nih.gov/articles/PMC6790599/

Title:	Social relations and presence of others predict bystander intervention: Evidence from violent incidents captured on CCTV	**by:**	National Center for Biotechnology Information (NCBI), National Library of Medicine (NLM), National Institutes of Health (NIH)
DOI:	10.1002/ab.21853	**Date:**	2019 Jul 29
Website:	PubMed Central (PMC)	**Publisher:**	Aggressive Behavior

[s25] - https://pmc.ncbi.nlm.nih.gov/articles/PMC6856396/

Title:	Speak Up! Prosocial Intervention Verbalizations Predict Successful Bystander Intervention for a Laboratory Analogue of Sexual Aggression	**by:**	National Library of Medicine (NLM)/ National Institutes of Health (NIH)
DOI:	10.1177/1079063218821121	**Date:**	2019 Jan 9
Website:	PubMed Central (PMC)	**Publisher:**	SAGE Publications

[s26] - https://pmc.ncbi.nlm.nih.gov/articles/PMC3017348/

Author:	Nancy Eisenberg (Department of Psychology, Arizona State University) ; Natalie D Eggum (Department of Psychology, Arizona State University) ; Laura Di Giunta (Interuniversity Centre for Research in the Genesis and Development of Prosocial and Antisocial Motivations, "Sapienza" University of Rome)	**Title:**	Empathy-related Responding: Associations with Prosocial Behavior, Aggression, and Intergroup Relations
DOI:	10.1111/j.1751-2409.2010.01020.x	**Date:**	2010 Dec 1
Website:	PubMed Central (PMC)	**Publisher:**	Wiley-Blackwell

[s27] - https://pmc.ncbi.nlm.nih.gov/articles/PMC3353316/

Author:	Ching Man Lam, Department of Social Work, The Chinese University of Hong Kong, Hong Kong	**Title:**	Prosocial Involvement as a Positive Youth Development Construct: A Conceptual Review
DOI:	10.1100/2012/769158	**Date:**	2012 Apr 30
Website:	PubMed Central (PMC)	**Publisher:**	The Scientific World Journal

[s28] - https://pmc.ncbi.nlm.nih.gov/articles/PMC4768593/

Author:	Zlatka Rakovec-Felser	**Title:**	Domestic Violence and Abuse in Intimate Relationship from Public Health Perspective
DOI:	10.4081/hpr.2014.1821	**Date:**	2014 Oct 22
Website:	PubMed Central (PMC)	**Publisher:**	PubMed Central (PMC)

[s29] - https://pmc.ncbi.nlm.nih.gov/articles/PMC5861012/

Author:	Danielle S Berke (University of Georgia, Athens, GA, USA)Dennis E Reidy (Centers for Disease Control and Prevention, Atlanta, GA, USA) Brittany Gentile (University of Georgia, Athens, GA, USA)Amos Zeichner (University of Georgia, Athens, GA, USA)	**Title:**	Masculine Discrepancy Stress, Emotion-Regulation Difficulties, and Intimate Partner Violence
DOI:	10.1177/0886260516650967	**Date:**	2016 May 24
Website:	PubMed Central (PMC)	**Publisher:**	Journal of interpersonal violence

[s30] - https://pmc.ncbi.nlm.nih.gov/articles/PMC11845222/

Title:	You-talk in young adult couples' conflict: Family-of-origin roots and adult relational aggression sequelae	**by:**	University of Virginia
DOI:	10.1177/02654075241270998	**Date:**	2024 Aug 5
Website:	PubMed Central (PMC)	**Publisher:**	PubMed Central (PMC)

[s31] - https://pmc.ncbi.nlm.nih.gov/articles/PMC2642009/

Author:	Heidemarie K Laurent (Oregon Social Learning Center, Eugene); Hyoun K Kim (Oregon Social Learning Center, Eugene); Deborah M Capaldi (Oregon Social Learning Center, Eugene)	**Title:**	Interaction and Relationship Development in Stable Young Couples: Effects of Positive Engagement, Psychological Aggression, and Withdrawal
DOI:	10.1016/j.adolescence.2007.11.001	**Date:**	2007 Dec 27
Website:	PubMed Central (PMC)	**Publisher:**	Journal of adolescence

[s32] - https://pmc.ncbi.nlm.nih.gov/articles/PMC8206473/

Author:	Rosa Isabel Rodrigues (Instituto Superior de Gestão, Lisbon, Portugal), Paula Lopes (Instituto Superior de Gestão, Lisbon, Portugal), Miguel Varela (Instituto Superior de Gestão, Lisbon, Portugal)	**Title:**	Factors Affecting Impulse Buying Behavior of Consumers
DOI:	10.3389/fpsyg.2021.697080	**Date:**	2021 Jun 2
Website:	PubMed Central (PMC)	**Publisher:**	Frontiers Media SA

[s33] - https://obssr.od.nih.gov/sites/obssr/files/Social-and-Behavioral-Theories.pdf

Title:	Social and Behavioral Theories	**by:**	Office of Behavioral and Social Sciences Research (OBSSR)
Date:	2014	**Website:**	Office of Behavioral and Social Sciences Research (OBSSR)
Publisher:	National Institutes of Health (NIH)		

[s34] - https://pmc.ncbi.nlm.nih.gov/articles/PMC7424041/

Title:	The Therapeutic Community: A Unique Social Psychological Approach to the Treatment of Addictions and Related Disorders	**by:**	National Library of Medicine (NLM), National Center for Biotechnology Information (NCBI)
DOI:	10.3389/fpsyt.2020.00786	**Date:**	2020 Aug 6
Website:	PubMed Central (PMC)	**Publisher:**	National Library of Medicine (NLM)

[s35] - https://pmc.ncbi.nlm.nih.gov/articles/PMC3603687/

Author:	Patricia G Devine, Patrick S Forscher, Anthony J Austin, William T L Cox	**Title:**	Long-term reduction in implicit race bias: A prejudice habit-breaking intervention
DOI:	10.1016/j.jesp.2012.06.003	**Date:**	2012 Nov
Website:	PubMed Central (PMC)	**Publisher:**	National Library of Medicine (NLM), National Institutes of Health (NIH)

[s36] - https://pmc.ncbi.nlm.nih.gov/articles/PMC2219858/

Author:	Diana Burgess (Center for Chronic Disease Outcomes Research, Veterans Affairs Medical Center; Department of Medicine, University of Minnesota) ; Michelle van Ryn (Center for Chronic Disease Outcomes Research, Veterans Affairs Medical Center; Department of Family Medicine and Community Health, University of Minnesota); John Dovidio (Department of Psychology, Yale University); Somnath Saha (Section of General Internal Medicine, Portland Veterans Affairs Medical Center and Department of Medicine, Oregon Health & Science University)	**Title:**	Reducing Racial Bias Among Health Care Providers: Lessons from Social-Cognitive Psychology
DOI:	10.1007/s11606-007-0160-1	**Date:**	2007 Mar 3
Website:	PubMed Central (PMC)	**Publisher:**	Springer

[s37] - https://pmc.ncbi.nlm.nih.gov/articles/PMC4090110/

Author:	Martin D Ruck, Henry Park, Melanie Killen, David S Crystal	**Title:**	Intergroup Contact and Evaluations of Race-Based Exclusion in Urban Minority Children and Adolescents
by:	PubMed Central (PMC)	**DOI:**	10.1007/s10964-010-9600-z
Date:	2010 Nov 4	**Website:**	PubMed Central (PMC)
Publisher:	National Library of Medicine (NLM)		

[s38] - https://pmc.ncbi.nlm.nih.gov/articles/PMC5311039/

Author:	Yuanyuan Shi (Beijing Key Lab of Applied Experimental Psychology, School of Psychology, Beijing Normal University, Beijing, China); Jianning Dang (Beijing Key Lab of Applied Experimental Psychology, School of Psychology, Beijing Normal University, Beijing, China); Wenwen Zheng (Beijing Key Lab of Applied Experimental Psychology, School of Psychology, Beijing Normal University, Beijing, China); Li Liu (Beijing Key Lab of Applied Experimental Psychology, School of Psychology, Beijing Normal University, Beijing, China)	**Title:**	Dual Identity and Prejudice: The Moderating Role of Group Boundary Permeability
by:	Beijing Normal University	**DOI:**	10.3389/fpsyg.2017.00195
Date:	2017 Feb 16	**Website:**	PubMed Central (PMC)
Publisher:	Frontiers in Psychology		

Image Sources

Unlisted images are either self-created or were acquired with appropriate license. All rights are reserved for these images.

For all other images listed here:
None of the images were modified, only the resolution was adjusted. In the eBook version, the images were compiled into numbered collages. All images remain subject to their original license and are used according to their respective license terms. If you discover any attribution errors or other discrepancies, please contact us.

Date of final image review: 2025-07-03.

Used License

CC0 http://creativecommons.org/publicdomain/zero/1.0/deed.en

Image Credits

[i1] - 001_001_002_image_fomo.jpeg
https://upload.wikimedia.org/wikipedia/commons/6/68/Screen_time.jpg
Date: 2018-10-01 **by:** Almaty
Artist: Rawpixel **License:** CC0

[i2] - 001_002_002_image_image.jpeg
https://upload.wikimedia.org/wikipedia/commons/5/58/Mask_Diabo_of_Portugal_used_on_folk_fest_and_rituals.jpg
Date: 2019-12-23 **by:** Wilfredor
Artist: Wilfredo Rafael Rodriguez Hernandez **License:** CC0

[i3] - 001_002_003_image_kleiderordnung.jpeg
https://upload.wikimedia.org/wikipedia/commons/5/55/Picture_of_dress_code_sign_outside_St_Joseph_TML_Primary_School.jpg
Date: 2024-12-08 **by:** 999real
License: CC0

[i4] - 001_003_001_image_einstellungsaenderung.jpeg
https://upload.wikimedia.org/wikipedia/commons/1/10/MRI_anterior_cingulate.png
Date: 2011-09-08 **by:** Geoff B Hall
License: CC0

[i5] - 001_003_002_image_footinthedoortechnik.jpeg
https://upload.wikimedia.org/wikipedia/commons/f/f4/Foot_in_the_door.jpg
Date: 2019-09-04 **by:** Ambrosia10
Artist: Siobhan Leachman **License:** CC0

[i6] - 002_001_003_image_doktortitel.jpeg
https://upload.wikimedia.org/wikipedia/commons/3/32/Georg_Bredig%27s_doctoral_diploma_-_DPLA_-_16886dc7bdda51bec10e1a5afd3bbfd9.jpg

Date:	1894	**by:**	DPLA bot
Artist:	Universität Leipzig (1409-1953)	**License:**	Public domain

[i7] - 002_001_003_image_luxusauto.jpeg
https://upload.wikimedia.org/wikipedia/commons/5/53/Luxury_Vehicle_Resort_%28Unsplash%29.jpg

Date:	2017-04-14	**by:**	Fae
Artist:	peterbroomfield	**License:**	CC0

[i8] - 002_002_001_image_autonomie.jpeg
https://upload.wikimedia.org/wikipedia/commons/8/8b/Keep_Out_Sign.jpg

Date:	2021-02-26	**by:**	MarkBuckawicki
License:	CC0		

[i9] - 002_002_001_image_konformitaetsdruck.jpeg
https://upload.wikimedia.org/wikipedia/commons/1/1e/USMC-110805-M-0992R-323.jpg

Date:	Taken	**by:**	Slick-o-bot
License:	Public domain		

[i10] - 002_002_001_image_nonkonformitaet.jpeg
https://upload.wikimedia.org/wikipedia/commons/0/06/Alok_Vaid-Menon_with_Flowers.jpg

Date:	2018-03-15	**by:**	Tamieparkersong
Artist:	Eivind Hansen	**License:**	CC0

[i11] - 002_003_003_image_vieraugengespraech.jpeg
https://upload.wikimedia.org/wikipedia/commons/7/70/Barack_Obama_has_a_private_conversation_with_House_Speaker_Nancy_Pelosi%2C_2009.jpg

Date:	Taken	**by:**	Vanished Account Byeznhpyxeuztibuo
Artist:	The White House	**License:**	Public domain

[i12] - 003_001_001_image_identifizierbarkeit.jpeg
https://upload.wikimedia.org/wikipedia/commons/4/4b/Signature-henri-d-orleans.jpg

Date:	2025-02-03	**by:**	Passepresent
License:	CC0		

[i13] - 003_001_001_image_gruppenkohaesion.jpeg
https://upload.wikimedia.org/wikipedia/commons/5/5f/US_Navy_090730-N-9418A-074_Senior_Chief_Ship%27s_Servicemen_Shawn_Johnson_and_Chief_Aviation_Machinist_Mate_Salvador_Reyes%2C_both_assigned_to_the_amphibious_assault_ship_USS_Essex_%28LHD_2%29%2C_participate_in_a_tug-of-war.jpg

Date:	Taken	**by:**	BotMultichillT
Artist:	U.S. Navy photograph by Mass Communication Specialist Seaman Taurean Alexander	**License:**	Public domain

[i14] - 003_001_001_image_teambuilding.jpeg
https://upload.wikimedia.org/wikipedia/commons/b/b0/US_Navy_040518-N-9693M-015_A_squad_of_Midshipmen_work_with_a_log_as_part_of_teamwork_training_during_Sea_Trials.jpg

Date:	Taken	**by:**	BotMultichillT
Artist:	U.S. Navy photo by Photographer's Mate 2nd Class Damon J. Moritz.	**License:**	Public domain

[i15] - 003_001_002_image_synergieeffekte.jpeg
https://upload.wikimedia.org/wikipedia/commons/a/a0/Synergy_trains%2C_Krasnaya_Presnya_depot.jpg

Date:	2017-03-17	**by:**	Xenotron
Artist:	Own work	**License:**	CC0

[i16] - 003_001_003_image_kognitive_belastung.jpeg
https://upload.wikimedia.org/wikipedia/commons/b/bf/Human_fatigue_study.jpg

Date:	2002-05-23	**by:**	Bomazi
Artist:	NASA Ames Research Center - Human Systems Integration Division	**License:**	Public domain

[i17] - 003_001_003_image_informationsueberflutung.jpeg
https://upload.wikimedia.org/wikipedia/commons/d/d4/Books%21_Books%21.jpg

Date:	2020-09-10	**by:**	Megan.hutchinson
License:	CC0		

[i18] - 003_002_001_image_plenum.jpeg
https://upload.wikimedia.org/wikipedia/commons/7/7e/ECAC-CEAC_36th_Plenary_%28triennial%29_Session_of_the_European_Civil_Conf%C3%A9rence%2C_Strasbourg_10_11_July_2018._%2828602800797%29.jpg

Date:	2018-07-10	**by:**	Edelseider
Artist:	ECAC ECAC	**License:**	CC0

[i19] - 003_002_003_image_stilles_brainstorming.jpeg
https://upload.wikimedia.org/wikipedia/commons/d/d6/WMNL-brainstorm_15_juni_2013-prioriteit.jpg

Date:	2013-06-15	**by:**	Romaine
License:	CC0		

[i20] - 003_003_001_image_soziale_identitaet.jpeg
https://upload.wikimedia.org/wikipedia/commons/c/c8/Democratic_Republic_of_Vietnam_identity_card_%281940%27s%29_01.jpg

Date:	2018-11-05	**by:**	Donald Trung
Artist:	The government of the Democratic Republic of Vietnam.	**License:**	Public domain

[i21] - 003_003_001_image_wirgruppe.jpeg
https://upload.wikimedia.org/wikipedia/commons/1/13/720th_Special_Tactics_Group_airmen_jump_20071003.jpg

Date:	2007-10-03	**by:**	Lycaon
Artist:	U.S. Air Force Airmen from the 720th Special Tactics Group out of Hurlburt Field, Fla., jump out of a C-130J Hercules aircraft during water rescue training above Choctawhatchee Bay. jpg	**License:**	Public domain

[i22] - 003_003_002_image_identifikation.jpeg
https://upload.wikimedia.org/wikipedia/commons/d/d0/BLM_Ryan_Lane_teaching_the_group_on_plant_identification_%287896121348%29.jpg

Date:	Taken	**by:**	OptimusPrimeBot
Artist:	USFWSAlaska	**License:**	Public domain

[i23] - 003_003_002_image_interdependenz.jpeg
https://upload.wikimedia.org/wikipedia/commons/f/ff/Screw_Coupling_used_in_Indian_Railways.jpg

Date:	28 October 2020	**by:**	Apurv013
Artist:	Apurba Biswas	**License:**	CC0

[i24] - 003_003_002_image_meilenstein.jpeg
https://upload.wikimedia.org/wikipedia/commons/f/f5/ArlingtonMAMilestoneBW.jpg

Date:	1933	**by:**	Magicpiano
Artist:	Historic American Buildings Survey	**License:**	Public domain

[i25] - 004_001_003_image_kindchenschema.jpeg
https://upload.wikimedia.org/wikipedia/commons/7/79/The_cute_dog%28poppy%29.jpg

Date:	2024-02-26	**by:**	Ranjithkanth Tamilselvan J
License:	CC0		

[i26] - 004_002_001_image_intervention.jpeg
https://upload.wikimedia.org/wikipedia/commons/4/46/SURFLANT_training_highlights_the_importance_of_bystander_intervention_150310-N-WJ261-003.jpg

Date:	Taken	**by:**	Fae
Artist:	Petty Officer 3rd Class amber odonovan	**License:**	Public domain

[i27] - 004_002_002_image_perspektivuebernahme.jpeg
https://upload.wikimedia.org/wikipedia/commons/b/b9/Taking_a_new_perspective_to_the_CN_Tower_%28Unsplash%29.jpg

Date:	2017-01-31	**by:**	Fae
Artist:	alx_andru	**License:**	CC0

[i28] - 004_002_002_image_gemeinnuetzigkeit.jpeg
https://upload.wikimedia.org/wikipedia/commons/5/53/Pre-Christmas_charity_action_%22Social_fridge_and_wardrobe%22_Information_banner_at_St._Antoni_Street%2C_Tomasz%C3%B3w_Mazowiecki%2C_Poland.jpg

Date:	2020-12-23	**by:**	WrS.tm.pl
Artist:	Warszawska rog Szerokiej w Tomaszowie Mazowieckim, w wojewodztwie lodzkim, PL, EU	**License:**	Public domain

[i29] - 004_003_001_image_impulskontrolle.jpeg
https://upload.wikimedia.org/wikipedia/commons/f/fb/Roasted-Marshmallow.jpg

Date:	2011-10-19	**by:**	Evan-Amos
License:	CC0		

[i30] - 004_003_001_image_kreislauf_der_gewalt.jpeg
https://upload.wikimedia.org/wikipedia/commons/9/9f/Israel_Palestine._The_eternal_cycle_of_violence._%2814665172593%29.jpg

Date:	2014-01-01	**by:**	Sentinel user
Artist:	EFFER LECEBE	**License:**	Public domain

[i31] - 004_003_002_image_zwerchfellatmung.jpeg
https://upload.wikimedia.org/wikipedia/commons/6/67/Paul_Von_Boeckman_advert.png

Date:	1913	**by:**	Veg Historian
Artist:	AnonymousUnknown author	**License:**	Public domain

[i32] - 005_001_003_image_partitionierung.jpeg
https://upload.wikimedia.org/wikipedia/commons/2/2a/US_Navy_090918-N-8560K-052_Machinist%27s_Mate_2nd_Class_Brannon_Kinsey%2C_assigned_to_the_aircraft_carrier_USS_George_H.W._Bush_%28CVN_77%29%2C_adds_coleslaw_to_a_tray_of_food_during_a_lunchtime_meal_at_St._Vincent_De_Paul_Catholic_Church.jpg

Date:	2009-09-18	**by:**	BotMultichillT
Artist:	U.S. Navy photo by Mass Communication Specialist 3rd Class Kasey Krall	**License:**	Public domain

[i33] - 005_002_001_image_lernen_durch_beobachtung.jpeg
https://upload.wikimedia.org/wikipedia/commons/f/ff/GoogleHangoutsMeeting.jpg

Date:	2015-05-20	**by:**	Raysonho
License:	CC0		

[i34] - 005_002_002_image_prokrastination.jpeg
https://upload.wikimedia.org/wikipedia/commons/6/62/Canva_-_Woman_Feeling_Emotional_Stress.jpg

Date:	2016-07-04	**by:**	Carovinc2
Artist:	MismibaTinasheMadando	**License:**	CC0

[i35] - 005_002_003_image_kompass.jpeg
https://upload.wikimedia.org/wikipedia/commons/5/59/Plastic-compass.jpg

Date:	2010-09-05	**by:**	Evan-Amos
License:	Public domain		

[i36] - 005_002_003_image_selbstverpflichtung.jpeg
https://upload.wikimedia.org/wikipedia/commons/3/37/Smokers_are_not_Selfish_Program_Commitment_to_quit_smoking_1.jpg

Date:	2025-05-27	**by:**	Wikiwebnepal
License:	CC0		

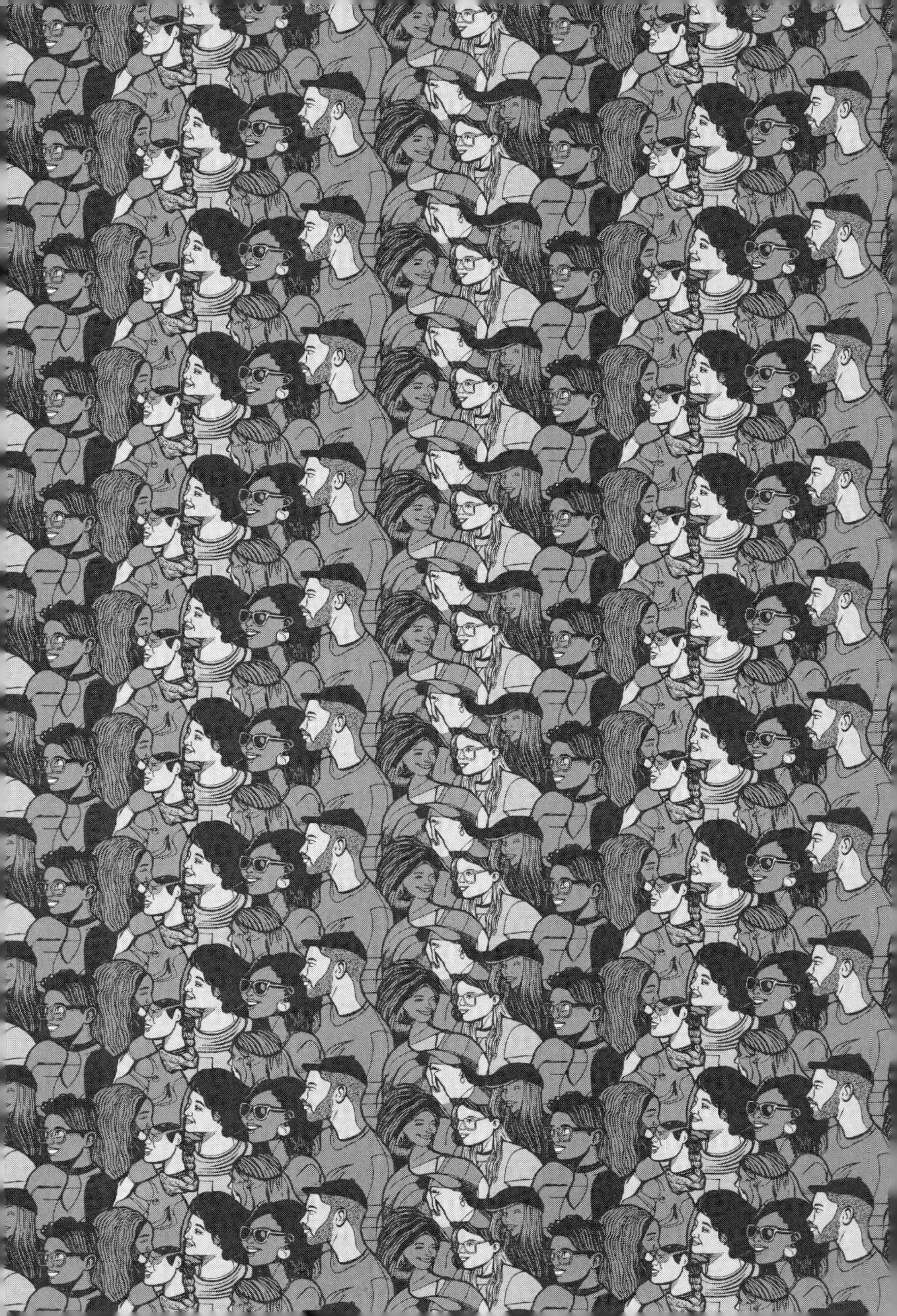

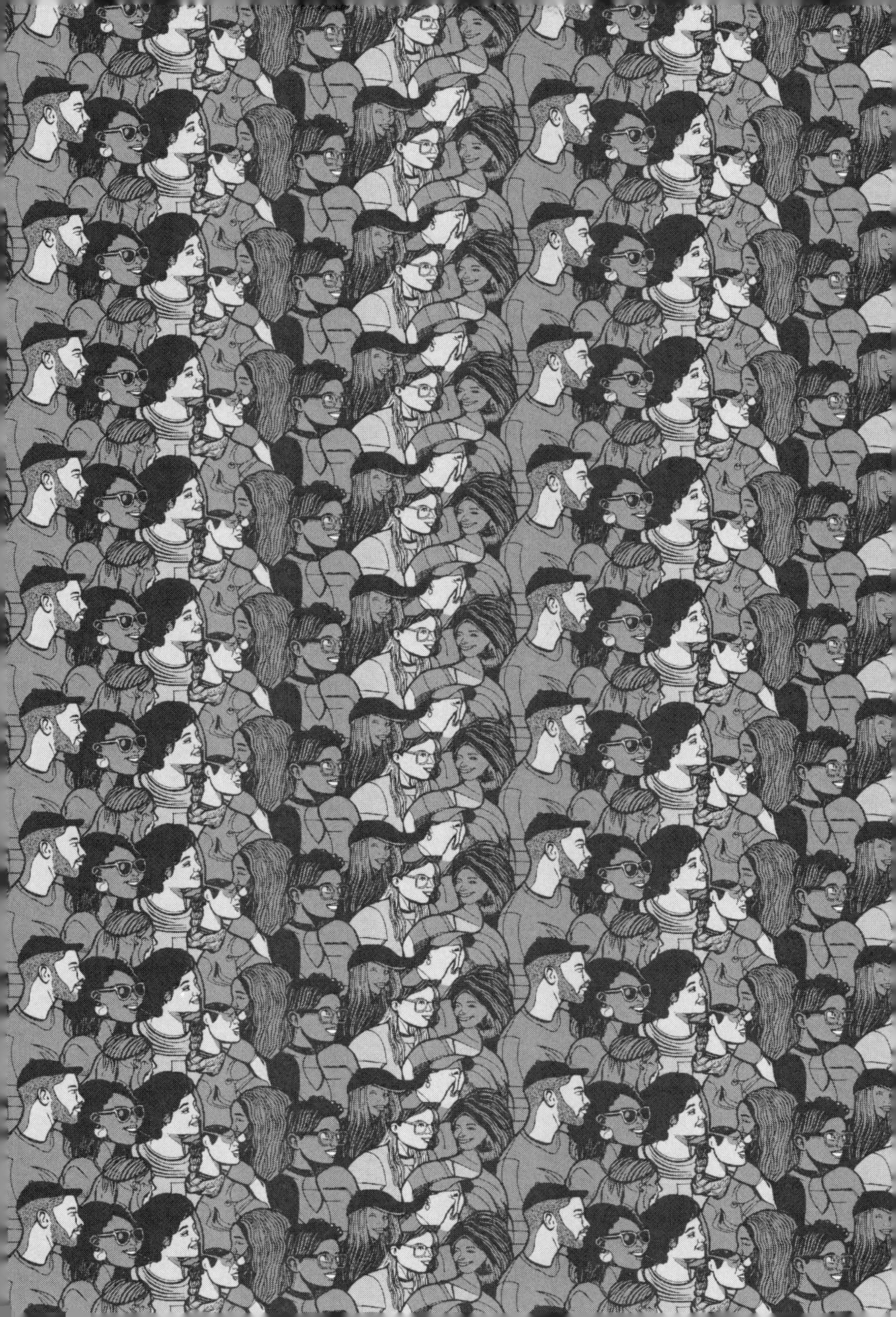

Made in United States
Orlando, FL
04 November 2026

90202667R10166